ENDOCRINE AND BIOLOGICAL THERAPY
OF
BREAST CANCER
INTO THE TWENTY-FIRST CENTURY

ENDOCRINE AND BIOLOGICAL THERAPY
OF
BREAST CANCER
INTO THE TWENTY-FIRST CENTURY

By
Kefah Mokbel MB, BS, MS, FRCS
*Consultant General Surgeon with a Special Interest in
Breast and Endocrine Surgery
St George's Hospital
London
and
Honorary Senior Lecturer in Biological Sciences at
Brunel University (Middlesex, UK)*

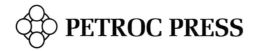 **PETROC PRESS**

Petroc Press, an imprint of LibraPharm Limited

Distributors
Plymbridge Distributors Limited, Plymbridge House, Estover Road,
Plymouth PL6 7PZ, UK

First edition 2001

Reprinted 2001

Published in the United Kingdom by
LibraPharm Limited
Gemini House
162 Craven Road
NEWBURY
Berkshire
RG14 5NR
UK

A catalogue record for this book is available from the British Library

ISBN 1 900603 19 5

Edited and Typeset by Martin Lister Publishing Services

Printed and bound by Cromwell Press Ltd, Trowbridge, UK

Contents

Introduction

Breast cancer remains the most common malignancy in women in the developed world. However, despite the slight increase in incidence over the last 20 years, breast cancer related mortality has been decreasing. This decline in mortality is partly due to screening and partly to the use of systemic chemotherapy and hormonal treatment. Traditionally, the development of a breast cancer drug has progressed from demonstrating efficacy in the advanced stage to demonstrating benefit in the adjuvant setting, and, in some examples, the clinical development has continued through demonstrating efficacy in the setting of breast cancer prevention.

Recent advances in molecular biology have enhanced our understanding of the mechanism of action of hormonal therapy and provided new targets for novel drugs.

This book provides a concise and up-to-date account of endocrine therapy for breast cancer. It covers historical development, basic physiology of female sex hormones, role of hormones in breast cancer aetiology, selective estrogen receptor modulators (SERMs), aromatase inhibitors, pure antiestrogens, ovarian ablation, promising biological therapies currently in development and chemoprevention. Key references have been provided throughout. The book also describes the recent advances in biological treatments targeting novel molecular components such as HER-2 oncogene, tyrosine kinases, matrix metalloproteinases and cyclo-oxygenase type II. Although the book aims to provide a concise and up-to-date medical guide to medical and surgical oncologists working in the field of breast cancer, it will also be valuable to general practitioners, postgraduate doctors in training and breast oncology nurses.

Kefah Mokbel FRCS
Consultant Breast Surgeon

Acknowledgements

I would like to thank all the contributors for being prompt, thorough and comprehensive. In particular, I would like to thank Mr C. Kouriefs MB, BS, MRCS, Miss J.C. Hu MB, BS, BSc, MBA, MRCS, Miss K. Kirkpatrick MB, BS, BSc, FRCS, Mr J. Benson MA, DM, FRCS and Dr P. L. Clarke PhD for their contribution.

I would like also to thank my wife Hanadi Kazkaz MD, MRCP for her encouragement during the inception and writing of this book.

Finally, acknowledgements would be incomplete without mentioning Mrs Lynn Frame and Miss Valmae Young who provided outstanding secretarial support.

Kefah Mokbel

1. The Physiological Basis

K. Mokbel

Introduction

The ovary is the predominant source of estrogens and progestins in non-pregnant, premenopausal women. In peripheral tissues such as muscle, skin and adipose tissue, estrogen is derived from adrenal androgens by the aromatase complex. In postmenopausal women, this represents the main source of estrogens. Small amounts of estrogens are also produced in the brain and male testis. During pregnancy, the feto-placental unit is the predominant source of estrogens and progestins.

Figure 1 illustrates the endometrial, ovarian and hormonal changes during the normal human menstrual cycle.

Estrogens

There are three natural human estrogens: 17β-estradiol (mainly ovarian), estriol (mainly placental) and estrone. Estrone is derived from androstenedione by aromatase and from 17β-estradiol by estradiol dehydrogenase and represents the main estrogen in postmenopausal women. Figure 2 demonstrates the pathway of estrogen synthesis. The target organs for estrogen and progesterone include the female reproductive tract, breasts, brain, adipose tissue, liver, kidneys, lungs and bone.

The gonadotrophin releasing hormone (GnRH) secreted by the hypothalamus stimulates the anterior pituitary to secrete follicle stimulating hormone (FSH) and luteinizing hormone (LH). These hormones stimulate the ovarian production of estrogen and progesterone. Positive and negative feedback loops regulate this hypothalamic–pituitary–

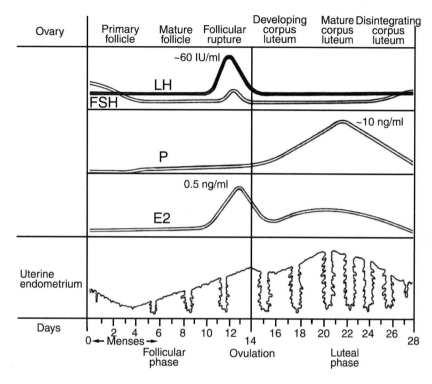

Figure 1 Endometrial, ovarian and hormonal changes during the normal human menstrual cycle. LH, luteinizing hormone; P, progesterone; FSH, follicle stimulating hormone; E2, estradiol

ovarian axis. In addition, pituitary ACTH (adrenocorticotrophic hormone) stimulates the adrenal cortex to produce androgens which are aromatized in peripheral tissues and converted into estrogens. The physiological actions of estrogens include:

(1) The development of secondary sex characteristics when the female enters puberty
(2) Fat deposition in the breasts, buttocks and thighs
(3) Increased stromal and ductal growth in the mammary glands
(4) Stimulation of cellular proliferation of uterine endometrium and stroma (if progesterone is absent)
(5) Thickening of vaginal mucosa and thinning of cervical mucosa
(6) Maintenance of bone mass
(7) Stimulation of cellular RNA and protein synthesis
(8) Stimulation of prolactin production by the pituitary gland

2

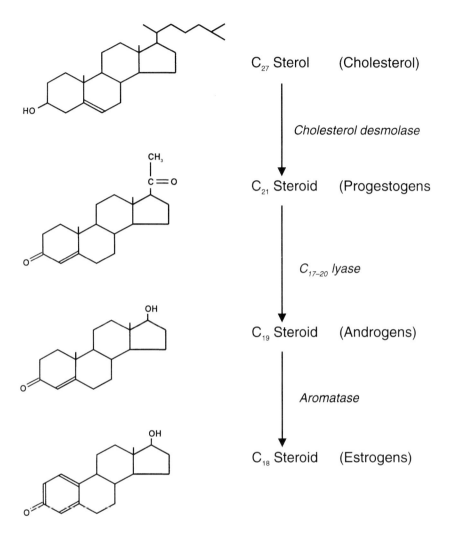

Figure 2 Pathway of estrogen biosynthesis

(9) Stimulation of growth at puberty
(10) Closure of epiphyses in the shafts of long bones
(11) Stimulation of hepatic synthesis of clotting factors (VII, VIII, IX and X), plasminogen, high density lipoproteins (HDL), sex-hormone binding globulin and thyroid binding globulin.

The pathological effects of prolonged estrogen exposure include increased risk of breast cancer and endometrial hyperplasia and carcinoma (in the absence of progesterone).

Progestins

Progesterone is the main natural progestin. Other progestins such as 20α-, 17α- and 20β-hydroxyprogesterone have weak progestational activity. The serum concentration of progesterone rises rapidly during the luteal phase of the menstrual cycle (Figure 1). The physiological effects of progesterone include:

(1)   Contribution to mammary gland development
(2)   Modulation of estrogen effects on the uterus resulting in secretory changes
(3)   Maintenance of pregnancy
(4)   Increased basal metabolic rate
(5)   Metabolic effects (e.g. ↑ LDL and ↓ HDL)

The Estrogen Receptor (ER)

Structure and Function[1]

The gene coding for the ER is located on chromosome 6 and is greater than 140 kb in length. The protein product of this gene is approximately 66 000 in molecular weight and contains 595 amino acids. It belongs to a super-family of nuclear receptor proteins. The ER protein contains six functional domains: the AB region is hypervariable and is thought to have constitutive transcriptional activation function (AF-1). The highly-conserved C domain is the most important as it has a DNA-binding function. This domain also includes two cysteine-rich zinc finger motifs and its amino acid sequence seems to determine the specific interactions between the receptor and the estrogen response elements (EREs). The D region is a variable hinge region that contains the sequences necessary for nuclear localization. The E domain functions include ligand binding, transcription activation function (AF-2) and the binding of heat shock protein (HSP). The ER is primarily located in the nucleus regardless of the presence of the ligand.

Although the receptor can passively diffuse into the cytoplasm, it is usually transported to the nucleus by an active process known as nucleocytoplasmic shuttle. In the inactive state, the ER is complexed with HSP which masks the DNA binding site. When estrogen binds to ER, the HSP is released causing changes in the ER structure and dimerization. This activated receptor binds avidly to EREs located in the vicinity of the target genes leading to enhancement of gene transcription by RNA polymerase. It is thought that ER–dimer–ERE complcx stabilizes pre-initiation proteins around RNA-polymerase thus activating the enzyme. AF-1, AF-2 and receptor interacting proteins (RIPs) also contribute to this activation process.

Measurement of ER

Determination of ER and progesterone receptor (PgR) is clinically important in patients with breast cancer, since the hormonal receptor status predicts prognosis and the likelihood of response to endocrine therapy[2,3]. The response rates to endocrine therapy in patients with ER- and PgR-positive tumours is approximately 70% compared with 10% in patients with ER- and PgR-negative tumours. Initially, the concentration of ER and PgR was determined using the dextran–charcoal method. In this method, a portion of the tumour is homogenized and centrifuged, then the supernatant is incubated with a known quantity of ^{3}H-labelled estrogen. The dextran is subsequently added to absorb unbound estrogen. The ^{3}H-labelled estrogen receptor complex remains in the supernatant and can be quantified by measuring the ^{3}H counts between the two tubes expressed in femtomoles per mg of protein. A tumour is considered to be ER or PgR positive if the receptor concentration exceeds 10 fmol/mg. The disadvantages of this method include the need for a large volume of fresh or frozen tumour tissue and the test is associated with a significant false negative rate in tumours that contain a small ER content. More recently, the ER and PgR contents have been measured by immunohistochemical techniques in which thin sections of formalin-fixed, paraffin-embedded tumour are exposed to monoclonal antibodies directed against the ER. The sections are then exposed to a secondary biotinylated antibody specific for the primary antibody. Subsequently, an avidin–peroxidase complex and a chromagen are added. The presence of ER is indicated by the appearance of a distinct colour. The percentage of stained cells and intensity of staining can be scored in order to quantify ER. The most widely accepted threshold for positivity is 10% which is equivalent to 10 fmol/mg protein as measured biochemically. Recent studies have shown that the new immunohistochemical method correlates well with biochemical ligand-binding techniques. However, immunohistochemistry has the advantage of speed, use of smaller portions of tumour and the ability to use formalin-fixed paraffin-embedded sections.

It should be pointed out that current methods effectively measure the ER-alpha subtype but not the ER-beta isoforms. This may explain why some ER-positive tumours are resistant to endocrine therapy.

ER Interactions

Estrogen-controlled genes include those that encode the PgR, proteases, transforming growth factor alpha (TGF-α), protein pS2 and thymidine kinase. Furthermore, over-expression of epidermal growth factor (EGF) and c-erbB2 seems to be associated with poor prognosis and ER negativity, and ER detection by immunohistochemistry does not perfectly correlate with its functional activity. In fact the presence of ER-regulated gene products such as PgR and pS2 proteins has been shown to be a better predictor of breast cancer prognosis than ER itself[4]. In familial breast cancer, Osin *et al.* have recently demonstrated that BRCA 1 tumours were less likely to be ER positive whereas BRCA 2 tumours had a similar ER-expression to that of sporadic breast cancer[5]. Continuous stimulation of ER with estradiol (E_2) seems to down-regulate ER expression via a negative feedback mechanism. Recent studies have also shown that methylation of the 5′ promoter of the gene blocks the transcription of ER mRNA in ER-negative cancer cells[6]. Protein kinase C which is over-expressed in ER-negative tumours seems to phosphorylate certain sites of the ER protein, rendering it inactive[7]. From a clinical standpoint, the interaction with PgR is the most important since PgR-negative tumours are less likely to respond to endocrine therapy. Retrospective studies have shown that 70% of PgR-positive tumours and 25% of PgR-negative tumours respond to endocrine therapy. More recently, the expression of c-erbB2 gene has been added to ER and PgR measurements in order to predict more precisely the response to hormonal treatment. A second human ER known as ER-beta has been recently identified[8]. Initial studies suggest that ER-beta positive tumours have favourable prognostic features and are likely to respond to hormonal therapy. However the independent predictive value of this recently described receptor remains to be established.

References

1. Rea DW, Parker MG. Structure and function of the estrogen receptor in relation to its altered sensitivity to oestradiol and tamoxifen. *Endocrine Related Cancer* 1995; **2**: 13–17.
2. Osborne CK. Steroid hormone receptors in breast cancer management. *Breast Cancer Res Treat* 1998; **51**: 227–238.
3. Chang J, Powles TJ, Allred DC *et al.* Prediction of clinical outcome from primary tamoxifen by expression of biological markers in breast cancer patients. *Clin Cancer Res* 2000; **6**: 616–621.
4. Iokaim-Liossi A, Karakitsos P, Markopoulos C *et al.* Expression of pS2 protein and estrogen and progesterone receptor status in breast cancer. *Acta Cytol* 1997; **3**: 713–716.
5. Osin P, Gusterson BA, Philp E *et al.* Predicted anti-oestrogen resistance in BRCA-associated familial breast cancers. *Eur J Cancer* 1998; **11**: 1683–1686.
6. Ottaviano YL, Issa JP, Parl FF *et al.* Methylation of the estrogen receptor gene CpG island marks loss of estrogen receptor expression in human breast cancer cells. *Cancer Res* 1994; **54**: 2552.
7. Tzukerman M, Zhang XK, Pfahl M. Inhibition of estrogen receptor activity by the tumour promoter 12-O-tetradeconylphorbol-13-acetate. A molecular analysis. *Mol Endocrinol* 1991; **5**: 1983–1992.
8. Jarvinen TA, Pelto-Huikko M, Holli K *et al.* Estrogen receptor beta is coexpressed with ER-alpha and PR and associated with nodal status, grade and proliferation rate in breast cancer. *Am J Pathol* 2000; **156**: 29–35.

2. Historical Development of Endocrine Therapy

C. Kouriefs and K. Mokbel

Over the last 20 years, there have been major advances in the medical management of breast cancer. However, breast cancer patients are still referred to surgical outpatients and are primarily managed and followed-up by surgeons. This is because despite all recent advances in medical therapies, surgery remains the mainstay of treating the primary tumour and the regional nodes.

In the mid-nineteenth century, Volkman proposed that breast cancer spreads downwards to the pectoral sheath, and therefore excision of the sheath would be necessary for cure. He, however, reported a 60% local recurrence rate and as a result, his theory did not fall into favour. In 1888, a Dr William Stewart of the Johns Hopkins Hospital proposed a new operative procedure for managing breast cancer, which he characterized as 'the complete method'[1]. He proposed an *en bloc* dissection of every tissue possibly affected by the tumour, including the pectoral muscles and lymph vessels in the axilla and up to the neck (Halsted radical mastectomy). Halsted's idea was based on Haudley's theory of centrifugal permeation, i.e. cancer cells permeate lymphatic channels in all directions thus reaching distant organs. In 1894, Halsted announced his first results:

> " ....in fifty cases operated upon by what we call a complete method, we have been able to trace only three local recurrences ...."

His (at the time) impressive results made his proposed procedure the dominant surgical treatment of breast cancer for many years.

Although the concept of excising all the areas involved by the cancer sounds very attractive, soon after Halsted's proposal of the 'complete method' it became clear that things were not so simple. Some tumours were too advanced at presentation to be excised. Tumours recurred locally or even distantly and the patients died after supposedly curative 'complete excision'. The need for new avenues to deal with weaknesses of 'complete excision' was first addressed by George T. Beatson, a surgeon at Glasgow Cancer Hospital.

> " .... *I have no doubt, it has fallen to the lot of every medical man to have been consulted from time to time by patients suffering from carcinoma so widely spread or so situated that it has been quite apparent that nothing in the way of operative measures could be recommended....*
>
> *Such cases naturally excite our sympathy but they also bring home to us the fact that once a case of cancer has passed beyond the reach of the surgeon's knife, our curative measures are practically nil and whether the case advances with giant strides or with slow and measured steps, the results are equally sure and fatal......* "

Dr G.T. Bateson was asked as a junior surgeon in the 1870s to take medical charge of a man whose 'mind was affected'. His duties, as he described, were at times exciting but never onerous. He therefore decided to start writing his M.D. thesis. He was influenced by a nearby sheep farm and took up the subject of lactation:

> "....*what suggested it to me was the weaning of the lambs in a large adjoining sheep farm soon after I went down to my patient......* "

During his thesis, he concluded that although the secretion of milk was undoubtedly affected by the nervous system, there seemed to be no nerve supply to the breast dedicated for that. Most importantly, he observed that the changes taking place in the breast during lactation were identical to those described in cancer of the mammary gland, namely epithelial proliferation. While collecting this information for his thesis, he learned that in some countries, farmers used to remove the ovaries of cows, after calving, if it was wished to keep up the supply of milk. If that was done, the cow would go on giving milk indefinitely. This information enabled him to give an explanation to his first observation that one organ could hold control over the secretions of another and separate organ. Unfortunately, he abandoned the subject of lactation for his thesis but never lost interest in it. When he settled and practised in Glasgow, in 1878, he was determined to give an answer to an attractive theory:

"I often ask myself, is cancer of the mamma due to some ovarian irritation as from some defective steps in the cycle of ovarian changes: and if so, would the cell proliferation be brought to a standstill or would the cells go on to the fatty degeneration seen in lactation were the cancer to be removed…"

In his article, 'treatment of inoperable cases of carcinoma of the mamma: suggestion for a new method of treatment, with illustrative cases'[2,3], he presented the very first three oophorectomies for advanced breast cancer. All three patients were premenopausal, one had a local recurrence after Halsted's mastectomy and the others had advanced disease. The first oophorectomy was performed on the June 8th, 1895. All three patients were started on thyroid tablets before proceeding to oophorectomy. Breast cancer did not respond to thyroid tablets and there was no mention of them in the conclusion. However, in all three cases, breast cancer responded favourably to oophorectomy and allowed Dr Beatson to conclude:

" my paper is headed 'the treatment of inoperable cases' and I am not in a position to replace the old plan of local removal – Which no doubt brings many disappointments, but has had of late years many encouraging results, by a new and untried method. All I feel is that there are grounds for the belief that the aetiology of the cancer lies not in the parasitic views but in an ovarian or testicular stimulus and that the whole subject requires careful working out…"

This was the very first suggestion of hormonal therapy for advanced breast cancer in premenopausal women. However, 120 years before George Beatson (1778), Percival Pott of St Bartholomew's Hospital reported a case of removal of normal ovaries in a 23-year-old woman, during the repair of bilateral inguinal hernia in which they became entrapped[4]….*"the patient enjoyed good health ever since…"* but ….*"Her breasts which were large are gone, nor has she ever menstruated since the operation which is now some years."*

In 1932, at St Bartholomew's Hospital, Sir Geoffrey Keynes, started his work on treating breast cancer with intense irradiation given off by radium chloride through platinum needles. He was the first to question the necessity for the so-far popular and promising Halsted's mastectomy.

> *"... Halsted's mastectomy entailed a gross mutilation of the patient's body in order to remove every scrap of tissue that might be infected by the spread of the disease through the lymphatic channels supposed to drain the breast ...."*

At the same time, there was a growing realization that cancerous growths quite early in their history could invade blood vessels and therefore cancer cells could spread to other parts of the body. Furthermore, it was realised that the normal lymphatic drainage of the breast was almost wholly by one main vessel passing to the axilla. The stream was interrupted by a group of lymph nodes which acted as a sieve to eliminate any foreign substances such as bacteria or cancer cells from reaching the circulation. When these nodes and the channels leading to them became blocked, new channels had to develop to relieve the pressure and cancerous permeation could proceed along these new channels. Haudley's centrifugal permeation was therefore considered as a terminal event and it was based on analysis of pathological specimens of patients with advanced lymphatic involvement.

Guided by his disbelief of Haudley's theory – the main justification for radical mastectomy – and by his work on irradiation of breast cancer, Sir Geoffrey Keynes, was the first to propose conservative surgery for breast cancer:

> *".... having satisfied myself that radium could be used successfully whether it might be used, perhaps in combination with conservative surgery for treating cancer of the breast in its early stages...."*

Conservative surgery was ignored until 1953, when Reginald Murby of St Bartholomew's hospital demonstrated that conservative surgical methods achieved as expected only a slight improvement in survival but a significant gain in quality of life. The move towards breast-conserving surgery was finally established in the 1980s. During that time, Veronesi *et al.* in Milan and Fisher *et al.* in USA conducted controlled studies to assess the safety of breast conserving surgery. Veronesi and colleagues compared Halsted mastectomy with quadrantectomy, surgical axillary clearance and radiotherapy to the remaining breast (QUART) and reported no survival differences[5]. Fisher *et al.* (B-06 trial) compared lumpectomy (clear margins) and axillary irradiation with total mastectomy and axillary clearance[6]. The authors again showed no survival differences between the two groups. Several trials have now shown no differences in mortality between breast conserving surgery and mastectomy but the local recurrence rate is slightly higher in the former.

Since George Beatson's paper in 1896, and for the first half of the 20th century, surgical ovariectomy became the surgical treatment of choice for advanced breast cancer in premenopausal women. The introduction of the less invasive ablation of ovarian function by irradiation in the 1920s and the recent development of synthetic hormones made surgical oophorectomy fall into temporary disfavour. In 1959, Patterson conducted the first randomized trial of ovarian ablation for early breast cancer, which may also be the first randomized trial for cancer treatment[7,8]. Several studies since have shown that ovarian ablation of functioning ovaries in early breast cancer improves long-term survival with significant benefit (at least in the absence of other adjuvant treatment) both in node-negative and node-positive breast cancer in premenopausal women[9].

In the second half of the 20th century, the potential role of the adrenal gland and the hypothalamic–pituitary axis, first in prostate and then in breast cancer, was recognized. Total surgical adrenalectomy in postmenopausal women and hypophysectomy (first in Sweden) in both pre- and postmenopausal women, were introduced for breast cancer. We have so far expanded on the history of the surgical endocrine management of breast cancer, but what about the more familiar medical endocrine therapy?

The first non-steroidal antiestrogen (MER 125) was introduced by Lerner and co-workers in 1958. However, tamoxifen or ICI 46,474 as it was first described, has taken all the credit in the management of breast cancer. It is one of the remarkable examples of a drug, which originally designed for a purpose that failed, and is now used successfully for another purpose. Tamoxifen was first synthesized in 1962, by Dr D. Richardson and it was shown to be an antifertility agent in rodents. When, however, it was tested on humans, it was found to induce ovulation and it was in fact used in some countries as an ovulation induction in subfertile women. By the end of the 1960s, the description of estrogen receptors in breast cancer reinforced the concept of estrogen dependence of breast cancer. The first clinical studies with tamoxifen for the management of advanced breast cancer in postmenopausal women were conducted at the Christie Hospital in Manchester in the late 1960s. The successful use of tamoxifen in advanced breast cancer encouraged animal studies, initially in Massachusetts in 1973 and then all over the world to describe in detail its tumourstatic action. In 1973, Nolvadex, the brand name of tamoxifen, was approved for the treatment of breast cancer by the Committee on Safety of Medicines in the UK. In 1977, similar approval was given in the USA for the treatment of advanced disease in postmenopausal women by the Food and Drug Administration. Since then, tamoxifen has been studied in clinical trials and used by millions of women as primary as well as adjuvant endocrine treatment in breast cancer. Tamoxifen has been shown to be beneficial in both pre- and postmenopausal women with node-negative and positive disease. What is of great interest, and remains to be determined by large randomized trials, is the use of tamoxifen as a chemopreventative agent in women at high risk of breast cancer.

The idea of chemoprevention of breast cancer goes back to 1936 when Lacassagne predicted that somehow we would be able to '.... prevent or antagonize the congestion of estrone in the breast....' Lacking any medical therapeutic agents, his observations were based on the effect of early oophorectomy on the development of breast cancer in a high-incidence strain of mice. Oophorectomy in young women would, however, be unacceptable as a preventative measure against breast cancer. The introduction of tamoxifen encouraged some animal model studies to assess the chemopreventative effect of tamoxifen. Such studies have shown that long-term tamoxifen treatment results in an initial classification of tamoxifen as an estrogen but within a few weeks the pharmacology changes and tamoxifen becomes an antiestrogen. Comparing tamoxifen with oophorectomy, the former seems to be a more effective mode of prevention with far fewer side-effects and humanly more acceptable when dealing with young women. In addition, tamoxifen mimics some of the physiological functions of estrogen by enhancing bone mineral density and lowering circulating cholesterol. The fact that tamoxifen use in stage I and II breast cancer led to a 50% reduction in contralateral tumours encouraged further research into its role in prevention. This led to the NSABP-P1 trial which confirmed a similar reduction in breast cancer risk in women at an increased risk of developing breast cancer[10]. Current research avenues for breast cancer prevention include the use of raloxifene. Women taking raloxifene for osteoporosis were shown to have a lower incidence of breast cancer (see Chapter 5). Tamoxifen and raloxifene are known as selective estrogen receptor modulators (SERMs).

Better understanding of the estrogen biosynthesis[11] in the 1960s opened other avenues for new medical endocrine treatments which have now replaced the surgical adrenalectomy and hypophysectomy of the mid-century. Estrogen synthesis requires the conversion of androstenedione to estrone by the aromatase enzyme system which involves three separate steroid hydroxylations utilizing an aromatase specific cytochrome P-450[12]. Aromatase activity in peripheral tissues such as fat, skin and muscle is the main source of estrogen in postmenopausal women and is gonadotrophin independent[13]. Aromatase inhibitors were therefore suggested as an endocrine therapy in postmenopausal women[14]. It was used in the clinical setting of breast cancer in post-menopausal women as an attempted medical adrenalectomy in 1973[15]. Aminoglutethimide with steroid replacement therapy was found to reduce plasma and urinary estradiol to levels similar to that achieved by surgical adrenalectomy and hypophysectomy[16]. The non-specific nature of aminoglutethimide with its associated side-effects stimulated interest in the development of other aromatase inhibitors, steroidal and non-steroidal, with different modes of action. Aromatase inhibitors are formally classified into 'suicide' and 'competitive' inhibitors. The suicide inhibitors (also known as aromatase inactivators), initially compete with the substrate for the enzyme and when they occupy the substrate-binding site, the enzyme acts upon them causing the development of irreversible covalent bonds. The advantage of that would be a long-lasting inhibition. On the other hand, competitive inhibitors bind reversibly to the enzyme. Aromatase inhibitors can be either steroidal or non-steroidal and have been shown to be effective as second line hormonal agents after tamoxifen failure[17–19]. Examples of modern aromatase inhibitors include anastrazole, letrozole and exemestane. In the 1980s, goserelin (Zoladex, AstraZeneca®), which is a decapeptide agonist at the LHRH receptor, was introduced as a potential treatment for breast cancer. LHRH analogues such as goserelin can reversibly suppress ovarian function in premenopausal women to castration levels. In the 1990s several studies demonstrated that Zoladex achieved an objective response in 36% of women with stage III and IV breast cancers. Furthermore, 50% of patients showed disease stabilization[20,21]. The role of these agents as an adjuvant treatment in premenopausal women with ER-positive early invasive breast cancer is currently being evaluated in clinical trials and the early results are promising. The enhanced understanding of the complex molecular biology of the ER and the growing evidence that estrogen promotes the development and growth of breast cancer have led to the development of a new class of drugs that block the ER with no agonist activity. This feature differentiates these pure antiestrogens from selective estrogen receptor modulators (SERMs) such as tamoxifen and raloxifene. Faslodex (ICI 182,780, AstraZeneca) is an example of such drugs and is currently being evaluated in the treatment of breast cancer[22]. Furthermore, Faslodex has been shown to down-regulate ER and has been therefore described as a selective ER down-regulator (SERD). It is possible that the high affinity of this drug for ER (90% of estradiol) may render ovarian suppression in premenopausal women unnecessary.

The Future

Several clinical trials evaluating the role of LHRH analogues as an adjuvant therapy for ER-positive early breast cancer and the role of pure antiestrogens such as Faslodex will report their results in the near future. The role of HER-2 overexpression in predicting tamoxifen failure in the adjuvant setting is likely to be clarified in the near future. Third-generation aromatase inhibitors are currently being compared head-to-head (e.g. anastrozole and letrozol) and with tamoxifen as a first-line therapy in postmenopausal women with early breast cancer. There is a growing body of evidence supporting their role as a first-line therapy for advanced breast cancer in postmenopausal women. The results of several studies will become available within the current decade. Furthermore, the role of aromatase inhibitors in the chemoprevention may be also evaluated.

Finally, the role of endocrine therapy for breast cancer will depend upon the relative success of novel biological therapies such as monoclonal antibodies and inhibitors of angiogenesis, metalloproteinases, tyrosine kinases, telomerase and growth factors receptors.

References

1. MacCallum WG. *William Stewart Halsted: Surgeon*. Baltimore, Johns Hopkins, 1930.

2. Beatson GT. Treatment of inoperable cases of carcinoma of the mamma: suggestion for a new method of treatment with illustrative cases. *Lancet* 1896; **2**:104–107.

3. Beatson GT. Treatment of inoperable cases of carcinoma of the mamma: suggestion for a new method of treatment with illustrative cases. *Lancet* 1896; **2**: 162–165.

4. Pott P. Ovarian hernia. *Chirurgical Works* 1775; 791–792.

5. Veronesi U, Zucali R, Del Vecchio M. Conservative treatment of breast cancer with QUART technique. *World J Surg* 1985; **9**: 676–681.

6. Fisher B, Bauer M, Margolese R *et al*. Five year results of a randomized clinical trial comparing total mastectomy and segmental mastectomy with or without radiation in the treatment of breast cancer. *N Engl J Med* 1985; **312**: 665–673.

7. Paterson R, Russell MH. Clinical trials in malignant disease. Part I *J Fac Radiol* 1958; **9**: 80.

8. Paterson R, Russell MH. Clinical trials in malignant disease. Part II *J Fac Radiol* 1958; **10**: 130–133.

9. Early Breast Cancer Trialists' Collaborative Group. Ovarian ablation in early breast cancer. Overview of the randomised trials. *Lancet* 1996; **348**: 1189–1196.

10. Fisher B, Costantino JP, Wickerham DL *et al*. Tamoxifen for the prevention of breast cancer: report of the National Surgical Adjuvant Breast and Bowel Project P-1 study. *J Natl Cancer Inst* 1998; **90**: 1371–1388.

11. Simpson ER, Merrill JC, Hellub AJ *et al*. Regulation of oestrogen biosynthesis by human adipose tissue cells. *Endocrine Rev* 1989; **10**: 136–148.

12. Richards JS, Hickey GJ, Chen SA *et al*. Hormonal regulation of oestradiol biosynthesis, aromatase activity and aromatase mRNA in rat ovarian follicles and corpora lutea. *Steroids* 1987; **50**: 393–409.

13. Santen RJ, Boucher AE, Santer SJ *et al*. Inhibition of aromatase as treatment of breast cancer in post menopausal women. *J Lab Clin Med* 1987; **109**: 278–289.

14. Cash R, Brough AJ, Cohen MN *et al*. Aminoglutethimide (Elipten-Ciba) as an inhibitor of adrenal steroidogenesis: mechanism of action and therapeutic trial. *J Clin Endocrinol Metab* 1967; **27**: 1239–1248.

15. Griffiths CT, Hall TC, Saba Z *et al*. Preliminary trial of aminoglutethimide in breast cancer. *Cancer* 1973; **32**: 31–37.

16. Stanten RJ, Worgul TJ, Samojlik E *et al*. A randomised trial comparing surgical adrenalectomy with aminoglutethimide plus hydrocortisone in women with advanced breast cancer. *N Engl J Med* 1981; **305**: 545–551.

17. Buzdar A, Jonat W, Howell A *et al*. Anastozole versus megestrol acetate in postmenopausal women with advanced breast cancer, mature survival data from the overview analysis of two phase III trials. Arimidex Study Group. *Cancer* 1998; **83**: 1142–1152.

18. Dombernowsky P, Smith I, Falkson G *et al*. Letrozole, a new oral aromatase inhibitor for advanced breast cancer: double-line randomised trial

showing a dose effect and improved efficacy and tolerability compared with megestrol acetate. *J Clin Oncol* 1998; **16**: 453–461.

19. Kaufmann M, Bajetta E, Dirix LY *et al.* Exemestane is superior to megestrol acetate after tamoxifen failure in postmenopausal women with advanced breast cancer: results of a phase III randomised double-blind trial. The Exemestane Study Group. *J Clin Oncol* 2000; **18**: 1399–1411.

20. Blamey RW, Jonat W, Kaumann M *et al.* Goserelin depot in the treatment of premenopausal advanced breast cancer. *Eur J Cancer* 1992; **28A**: 810–814.

21. Taylor CW, Green S, Dalton WS *et al.* Multicentre randomised clinical trials of goserelin versus surgical ovariectomy in premenopausal patients with receptor positive metastatic breast cancer. *J Clin Oncol* 1998; **16**: 993–999.

22. Diel P, Smolnikar K, Michna H. The pure antiestrogen ICI 182780 is more effective in the induction of apoptosis and down regulation of BCL-2 than tamoxifen in MCF-7 cells. *Breast Cancer Res Treat* 1999; **58**: 87–97.

3. Hormones and Mammary Carcinogenesis

K. Mokbel

Endogenous Hormones

Seven out of eight prospective studies of postmenopausal women reported an increased risk of breast cancer in association with elevated levels of estradiol[1-8]. An overall analysis of these studies shows that the relative risk is 2.3 (95% CI = 1.6–3.2) for women with highest levels relative to those with lowest serum estradiol. Such an observation has not been confirmed in premenopausal women[9,10], whose hormones show a wide physiological variation, thus complicating analysis.

Further evidence for the role of endogenous estradiol in the aetiology of breast cancer is also derived from the epidemiological studies showing that early menarche and late menopause are associated with an increased risk of developing the disease and from chemoprevention studies[10,11] which have demonstrated a significant reduction of breast cancer incidence in women at an increased risk. These trials used serum estrogen receptor modulators, namely tamoxifen[10] and raloxifene[11,12] which are known to have antiestrogenic activity in the breast.

The most likely mechanism mediating the carcinogenic effect of estrogens in the breast is the increased rate of mitosis in breast epithelial cells[13,14]. The risk of DNA mutations is increased in cells with high mitotic rates. There is increasing evidence that steroid hormones and growth factor signalling pathways cross-talk to reinforce each other's signalling[15]. Obesity in postmenopausal women is also known to increase breast cancer risk. The condition is associated with increased serum estradiol levels through increased activity of aromatase acting on androstenedione and estrone[16]. Obesity is also associated with reduced serum levels of sex hormone binding globulin[16]. Other endogenous hormones such as prolactin and insulin like growth factor I (IGF-I) have been found to be associated with an increased risk of breast cancer. Hankinson *et al.* reported that increased serum IGF-I was associated with increased risk of breast cancer in premenopausal women[17]. Hankinson and colleagues also showed that increased serum prolactin was associated with increased risk of breast cancer in postmenopausal women[18]. It is likely that these hormones interact with endogenous estrogens in mediating their effects on breast cancer risk. The effect of progesterone on breast cancer risk remains unclear.

Exogenous Hormones

In 1997, the Collaborative Group on Hormonal Factors in Breast Cancer published the results of their re-analysis, examining the effects of hormone replacement therapy (HRT) on breast cancer risk[19]. The results of this study were based on more than 160 000 women from 21 countries who participated in 51 different epidemiological studies over the past 25 years. These data represent more than 90% of the world's literature on the subject. The authors observed that among current and recent (those who stopped using HRT 1–4 years previously) users, the relative risk of having breast cancer diagnosed increased by a factor of 1.023 (95% CI = 1.011–1.036; 2p = 0.0002) for each year of use. For women who had used HRT for 5 years or longer, the relative risk was 1.35 (95% CI = 1.21–1.49; 2p = 0.00001). This increase in risk is equivalent to the effect on breast cancer risk of delaying the menopause. After 5 years of HRT cessation, there was no excess breast cancer in patients who had used HRT. In this analysis, only 12% of HRT users had been exposed to progesterones. However, a recent study reported that postmenopausal women taking combination HRT with estrogen and progesterone feared a greater risk of developing breast cancer than those taking estrogen alone[20]. Combination HRT increased breast cancer risk by 40% compared with 20% for estrogen only. However, the mode of replacement, continuous versus cyclic, was not controlled for and therefore further studies are required.

Although HRT increases the risk of developing breast cancer, there is no evidence that it increases breast cancer-related mortality. In a study of 984 women with breast cancer, Jernstrom *et al.* reported that HRT use was an independent predictor of longer survival[21]. Such observations are consistent with the recent findings of the Iowa Women's Health Study[22] which involved 37 105 women at risk of developing breast cancer. The authors observed that exposure to HRT was associated with an increased risk of invasive breast cancer with a favourable prognosis. The information should be borne in mind when assessing the benefits and risks of HRT.

Whether women who have been treated for breast cancer could be safely prescribed HRT remains open to question and requires prospective randomized clinical trials. However, there is no evidence that HRT use after 5 years of breast cancer treatment worsens outcome[23].

References

1. Garland CF, Friedlander NJ, Barrett-Connor E *et al.* Sex hormones and postmenopausal breast cancer: a prospective study in an adult community. *Am J Epidemiol* 1992; **135**: 1220–1230.
2. Helzlouer KJ, Alberg AJ, Bush TL *et al.* A prospective study of endogenous hormones and breast cancer. *Cancer Detect Prev* 1994; **18**: 79–85.
3. Toniolo PG, Levitz M, Zeleniuch-Jacquotte A *et al.* A prospective study of endogenous estrogens and breast cancer in post-menopausal women. *J Natl Cancer Inst* 1995; **87**: 190–197.
4. Berrino F, Muti P, Michel A *et al.* Serum sex hormone levels after menopause and subsequent breast cancer. *J Natl Cancer Inst* 1996; **88**: 291–296.
5. Dorgan JF, Longscope C, Stephenson HE Jr *et al.* Relation of prediagnostic serum estrogen and androgen levels to breast cancer risk. *Cancer Epidemiol Biomarkers Prev* 1996; **5**: 533–539.
6. Thomas HV, Key TJ, Allen DS *et al.* A prospective study of endogenous serum hormone concentration and breast cancer risk in postmenopausal women on the Island of Guernsey. *Br J Cancer* 1997; **76**: 401–405.
7. Hankinson SE, Willett WC, Manson JE *et al.* Plasma sex steroid hormone levels and risk of breast cancer in postmenopausal women. *J Natl Cancer Inst* 1998; **90**: 1292–1299.
8. Cauley JA, Lucas FL, Kuller LH *et al.* Elevated serum estradiol and testosterone concentrations are associated with a high risk for breast cancer. *Ann Intern Med* 1999; **130**: 270–277.
9. Thomas HV, Key TJ, Allen DS *et al.* A prospective study of endogenous serum hormone concentration and breast cancer risk in premenopausal women on the Island of Guernsey. *Br J Cancer* 1997; **75**: 1075–1079.
10. Fisher B, Constantino JP, Wickerham DL *et al.* Tamoxifen for prevention of breast cancer: Report of the National Surgical Adjuvant Breast and Bowel Project P-1 Study. *J Natl Cancer Inst* 1998; **90**: 1371–1388.

11. Cummings SR, Eckert S, Kreuger *et al.* The effect of raloxifene on the risk of breast cancer in postmenopausal women: results from the MORE randomised trial. *JAMA* 1999; **281**: 2189–2197.

12. Cauley J, Kruegger K, Eckert S *et al.* Breast cancer risk in postmenopausal women with osteoporosis is reduced with raloxifene treatment: extension of the MORE trial data to a median follow-up of 48 months. *Proc Am Soc Clin Oncol* 2000; **88a**: Abstr.356.

13. Anderson TJ, Ferguson DJP, Raab GM. Cell turnover in the 'resting' human breast: influence of parity contraceptive pill, age and laterality. *Br J Cancer* 1982; **46**: 376–382.

14. McManus MJ, Welsch CW. The effect of estrogen, progesterone, thyroxine and human placental lactogen on DNA synthesis of human breast ductal epithelium in athymic nude mice. *Cancer* 1984; **54**: 1920–1927.

15. Nicholson RI, Gee JMW. Oestrogen and growth factor cross-talk and endocrine insensitivity and acquired resistance in breast cancer. *Br J Cancer* 2000; **82**: 501–513.

16. Siiteri PK, McDonald PC. Role of extraglandular estrogen in human endocrinology In Geiger SR, Astwood EB, Greep RO, eds, *Handbook of Physiology*. Washington DC: American Physiological Society, 1973; **2**: 615–629.

17. Hankinson SE, Willett WC, Colditz GA *et al.* Circulating concentrations of insulin-like growth factor-I and risk of breast cancer. *Lancet* 1998; **351**: 1393–1396

18. Hankinson SE, Willett WC, Michaud DS. Plasma prolactin levels and subsequent risk of breast cancer in postmenopausal women. *J Natl Cancer Inst* 1999; **91**: 629–634.

19. Collaborative Group on Hormonal Factors in Breast Cancer. Breast cancer and hormone replacement therapy. Collaborative reanalysis of data from 51 epidemiological studies of 52705 women with breast cancer and 108411 women without breast cancer. *Lancet* 1997; **35**: 1047–1059.

20. Shchairer C, Lubin J, Troisi R *et al.* Menopausal estrogen and estrogen–progestin replacement therapy and breast cancer risk. *JAMA* 2000; **283**: 485–491.

21. Jernstrom H, Frenander J, Ferno M *et al.* Hormone replacement therapy before breast cancer diagnosis significantly reduces the overall death rate compared with never-use among 984 breast cancer patients. *Br J Cancer* 1999; **80**: 1453–1458.

22. Gapstur SM, Morrow M, Sellers TA. Hormone replacement therapy and risk of breast cancer with a favourable histology. Results of the Iowa Women's Health Study. *JAMA* 1999; **281**: 2091–2097.

23. Ursic-Vrscaj M, Bebar S. A case control study of hormone replacement therapy after primary surgical breast cancer treatment. *Eur J Surg Oncol* 1999; **25**: 146–151.

4. Tamoxifen

K. Mokbel and J. Benson

Introduction

Tamoxifen is the original example of a selective oestrogen receptor modulator (SERM) and is a functionally heterogeneous agent with mixed agonist and antagonist properties. Its principal action is to antagonize oestrogen at the level of cellular receptors, but ER independent modes of action exist[1]. Furthermore, the agonist properties of tamoxifen confer incidental clinical benefits on bone and the cardiovascular system, although such agonist activity may ultimately compromise anti-tumour action.

Tamoxifen (initially designated ICI 46474) is a triphenylethylene derivative in contrast to pure anti-oestrogens which are alkylamide analogues of oestradiol (Figure 1)[2]. Pure anti-oestrogens therefore lack the basic triphenylbutene core which defines the chemical structure of the triphenylethylene group of SERMs, although, in common with triphenylethylenes, they possess a side-chain with basic/polar groups which are essential for oestrogen antagonist properties. In consequence, they are devoid of agonist properties and the beneficial clinical sequelae which assume greater significance in a chemopreventive context and may partially provide the ethical justification thereof.

As a sex hormone antagonist, tamoxifen was initially developed as an oral contraceptive agent, although Walpole investigated the role of triphenylethylenes in breast cancer in the 1940s[3]. However, its failure in this capacity was eclipsed by its successful application in the treatment of breast cancer. Tamoxifen was first investigated as an alternative form of hormone manipulation in patients with advanced breast cancer[4,5]. Cole and colleagues undertook a preliminary study involving 46 post-menopausal patients with advanced breast cancer, of whom

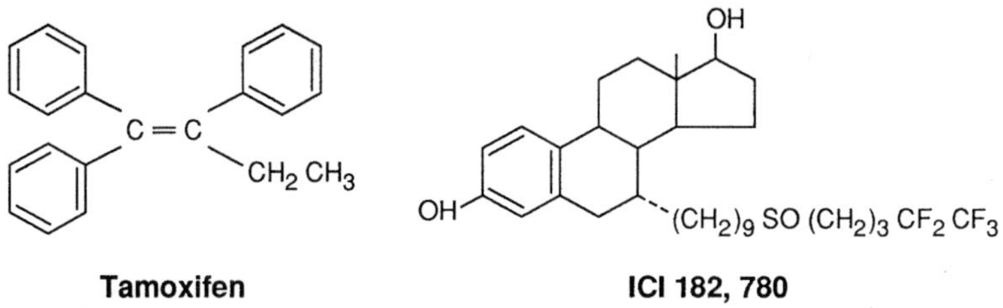

Tamoxifen   **ICI 182, 780**

Figure 1 Structure of tamoxifen which is a non-steroidal triphenylethylene derivative, and the 'pure' anti-oestrogen ICI182,780 which is an alkylamide derivative of oestrogen. Both molecules possess a basic/polar side-chain which confers anti-oestrogen activity

one-quarter responded to treatment with tamoxifen. This agent was subsequently employed in the adjuvant setting, thus heralding the era of widespread tamoxifen use for early-stage breast cancer. Clinical trials of tamoxifen as adjuvant therapy were initiated in the 1970s and improvements in disease-free and overall survival were most apparent in post-menopausal, node-positive patients with ER-rich tumours These findings were consistent with its activity profile in advanced disease[6]. With further analysis involving increased numbers of patients and longer follow-up, tamoxifen was found to be beneficial in other subgroups, including node-negative patients and those with 'ER-poor' tumours[7–9].

Tamoxifen is metabolized to several products which have anti-tumour activity. The principle metabolites are *N*-desmethyltamoxifen and the 4-OH-derivative which is metabolically active. However, experiments investigating the functional profiles of tamoxifen and related triphenyl-ethylenes in an *in vitro* model have shown 4-OH-tamoxifen to be no more active than the parent compound[10]. Furthermore, this 4-OH derivative forms DNA adducts and remains potentially mutagenic with a relatively long half-life. Other analogues of tamoxifen such as raloxifene and idoxifene possess a modified alpha-phenyl ring which prevents adduct formation[11]. This not only reduces their carcinogenic effects but also attenuates ureterotrophic activity. These compounds represent second-generation SERMs and have a modified agonist profile with retention of beneficial effects upon bone and the cardiovascular system. They are therefore highly attractive as potential successors to tamoxifen for adjuvant treatment and chemoprevention of breast cancer. Nonetheless, the anti-tumour efficacy of raloxifene has been questioned, despite an overview of randomized studies of raloxifene revealing a 58% reduction in breast cancer risk ($p \leq 0.0001$)[12]. Raloxifene is currently being compared with tamoxifen for chemoprevention of breast cancer in high risk post-menopausal women (Study of Tamoxifen and Raloxifene (STAR) trial).

Mechanisms of Action

Tamoxifen exerts its antitumour effects through several mechanisms[1,13], although ER-dependent pathways dominate.

ER-dependent Mechanisms

Anti-oestrogens antagonize the action of oestrogen and act as competitive inhibitors for the ligand binding site of the ER. The ER–tamoxifen complex therefore abrogates the biological function of oestrogen and prevents expression of oestrogen-regulated genes. Tamoxifen and related triphenylethylenes are 'impure' anti-oestrogens and can invoke an attenuated transcriptional response by permitting dimerization of ER–tamoxifen complexes and some DNA-binding[14]. However, transcription is incomplete due to imperfect association of co-activators with the ER–tamoxifen complex (Figures 2 and 3).

Enzyme Inhibition

Tamoxifen inhibits the enzyme protein kinase C (PKC) in a sub-cellular enzyme system[15]. This protein kinase is both calcium and phospholipid dependent and is activated by diacylglycerol (a product of inositol phospholipid hydrolysis), together with tumour-promoting phorbol esters[16]. Tamoxifen appears to indirectly prevent enzyme activation by interacting with the phospholipid moiety[17]. The role of PKC as a signal transducer in breast cancer cells, and the significance of any inhibition of PKC by tamoxifen remains unclear.

Another enzyme inhibited by tamoxifen is calmodulin-dependent cAMP phosphodiesterase (CPD)[18]. ER and calmodulin may be involved in coupled-signalling pathways controlling hormone-dependent cellular proliferation[19]. Inhibition of CPD may only be of significance in ER-positive cells, as binding of tamoxifen to the ER is necessary for inhibitory effects upon calmodulin.

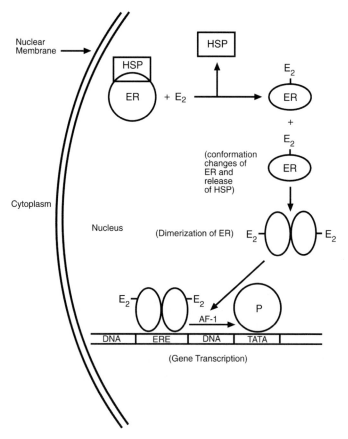

Figure 2 Mechanism of action of 17β-estradiol (E2). ER, estrogen receptor; HSP, heat shock protein; ERE, estrogen response elements; TATA, nucleotide sequence that indicates the starting point of transcription; P, pre-initiation complex

Local induction of TGF-β

There is evidence for induction of the inhibitxory growth factor trans-forming growth factor β (TGF-β) in response to a variety of therapeutic agents, including tamoxifen. The role of TGF-β in mediating a response to a therapeutic intervention is often difficult to distinguish from its role in carcinogenesis *per se*[20]. Furthermore, there is much controversy over the source of any pharmacologically-induced TGF-β, which may be of either epithelial or stromal origin. It has been proposed that tamoxifen may directly stimulate fibroblasts to produce and secrete TGF-β which can act in a negative paracrine manner upon neighbouring epithelial

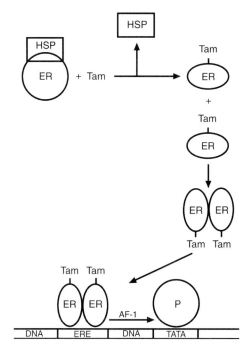

Figure 3 Mechanism of action of tamoxifen (Tam). The ER–Tam dimer interacts with ERE resulting in antiestrogenic effects if gene transcription is completely controlled by activation function 2 (AF-2) and estrogenic effects if gene transcription is purely controlled by AF-1. Tamoxifen effects are mixed if AF-1 and AF-2 control gene transcription

cells[10] (Figure 4). Tamoxifen induces secretion of TGF-β between 3- and 30-fold in foetal fibroblasts *in vitro*[10] and stromal induction of TGF-β occurs in both ER-positive and ER-negative breast cancer patients following 3 months of primary tamoxifen therapy[21]. Moreover, increased synthesis of TGF-β in response to tamoxifen has been reported in primary cultures of breast tumour fibroblasts *in vitro*[22].

Anti-angiogenic Effects

Tumour vessel count/grade has been correlated with lymph node status and survival in breast cancer, with higher vessel counts being associated with poorer clinical outcome[23,24]. Tamoxifen has been demonstrated to have anti-angiogenic activity in a chick chorioallantoic membrane model[25] and can reduce endothelial cell proliferation in the early stages of vascular regeneration following trauma[26]. Inhibition of angiogenesis represents a potentially important anti-tumour strategy, and anti-angiogenic agents are under clinical investigation as adjuvants.

Systemic Effects

Tamoxifen has a variety of systemic effects which may contribute to its anti-tumour activity. In addition to local induction of TGF-β, there is evidence for modulation of both systemic and local levels of insulin-like growth factors (IGF I and IGF II)[27,28]. These are potent mitogens for breast cancer cells which express type I IGF receptors for which both IGF I and IGF II are functional ligands. Adjuvant tamoxifen therapy is associated with a 30% decrease in serum IGF I levels[27]. Breast tumour epithelium may participate in a positive paracrine pathway whereby fibroblasts are stimulated by epithelial cells to secrete insulin-like growth factors which stimulate proliferation of adjacent epithelium (Figure 4). Tamoxifen also augments levels of IGF-binding proteins, thus sequestering these agents and reducing their biological activity. Furthermore, this agent may exert other effects via indirect mechanisms; metastatic and invasive potential may be suppressed by down-regulation of oestrogen-controlled proteases and immuno-modulation may be indirectly influenced by changes in growth factor expression.

Tamoxifen for Early Invasive Carcinoma

The most recent overview of randomized controlled trials of tamoxifen therapy confirms the clinical indications for this agent as an adjuvant treatment for early breast cancer[29]. This meta-analysis evaluated 30 000 patients of whom 18 000 were ER positive and 12 000 were of unknown ER status (of whom two-thirds were estimated to be ER positive). The overall proportional reduction in annual odds of local recurrence and mortality at 10 years was 47% and 26% respectively after 5 years of tamoxifen. This analysis excluded 8000 patients with 'ER-poor' tumours most of whom received only 1–2 years of treatment with only 12% receiving 5 years of tamoxifen. It therefore remains unclear whether more prolonged therapy in this group (about 5 years) may yield greater benefits, especially for post-menopausal patients. The clinical benefits of tamoxifen increased progressively with longer

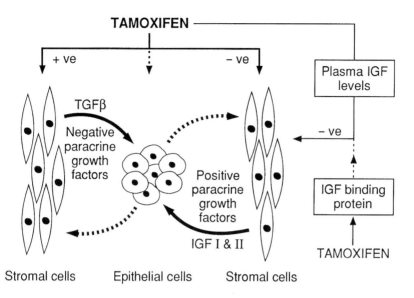

TAMOXIFEN

Stromal cells   Epithelial cells   Stromal cells

Figure 4 Unifying schema showing how tamoxifen may modulate growth factor levels by several mechanisms involving stimulation or suppression of positive and negative growth factors derived from either stromal or epithelial cells. Thus tamoxifen may directly stimulate either stromal or epithelial cells to enhance secretion of TGF-β. Conversely it can act upon the same cells to suppress production of positive growth factors such as IGF I and IGF II. Changes in levels of binding proteins can control bioavailability of growth factors (Reprinted with permission from: Benson JR, Baum M, Colletta AA. In deVita, Hellman, Rosengerg, eds. *Biologic Therapy of Cancer*, 2nd edn. 1995: 817–828. Copyright Lippincott–Raven Publishers)

duration of tamoxifen therapy and were greatest in patients with tumours expressing high levels of ER. By contrast, the proportional reduction in mortality for ER-poor tumours was only 6%. Up to one-fifth of ER-poor tumours contain functional progesterone receptor (PgR) and this may confer a degree of hormonal responsiveness which differs from tumours with dual negativity for ER and PgR for which there is minimal benefit from adjuvant tamoxifen therapy. The relative risk reductions in relapse were similar for pre- and post-menopausal women and there was no statistically significant difference in proportional mortality reductions between node-negative and node-positive patients, although absolute benefits were greater for the latter.

The survival benefits of tamoxifen therapy persisted beyond 5 years after cessation of tamoxifen; proportional risk reductions over the subsequent 4 years were comparable to the initial 5 year period. Furthermore, tamoxifen therapy reduced the incidence of contralateral breast cancer in proportion to duration of therapy, and for 5 years of treatment this reduction was almost 50%. Tamoxifen therapy is associated with an increased incidence of endometrial carcinoma which is approximately 4-fold following 5 years of therapy. However, endometrial tumours invariably present at an early stage when treatment is highly effective.

Tamoxifen and Advanced Breast Cancer

The overall response rate in patients with metastatic disease is approximately 35% with a further 20% showing disease stabilization[30]. The response rate depends on ER status with 45% of patients with ER-positive tumours responding to treatment compared with 10% of ER-negative patients[31]. The median duration of response is 12 months. Although tamoxifen demonstrated similar response rates to surgical oophorectomy in the treatment of premenopausal women with metastatic breast cancer[32], the SWOG study[33] reported a lower response rate among premenopausal women (24 vs 57%). In women with locally-advanced ER-positive breast cancer, tamoxifen can be used as a neoadjuvant therapy in order to reduce the size of the tumour and render it amenable to breast conserving surgery. Furthermore, frail elderly patients with locally-advanced breast cancer can be treated with tamoxifen alone, achieving good local control in approximately 35% of cases.

Tamoxifen and DCIS

Fisher and colleagues reported the findings of the NSABP-24 study in 1999. A total of 1804 women with DCIS (including those with positive resection margins) undergoing local excision and radiation treatment (50 Gy) were randomized to receive either tamoxifen (20 mg daily) for 5 years or placebo. Patient characteristics were matched for the two groups which each contained 902 patients. The cumulative incidence of all breast cancer events at 5 years was 13.4% and 8.2% for placebo and tamoxifen groups respectively (Figure 5). Overall survival was similar for both groups (97%). The benefits of tamoxifen were significant irrespective of margin status and the presence of comedonecrosis.

Ipsilateral breast

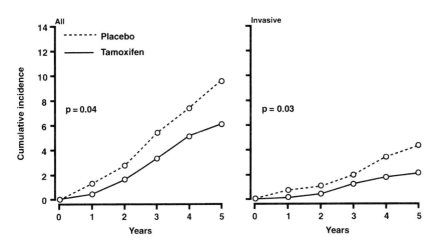

Figure 5 The cumulative incidence of **all** and **invasive** cancer events in the ipsilateral breast after breast conserving surgery and adjuvant radiotherapy for DCIS (*n* = 1804). Findings of the NSABP-B24 trial

Tamoxifen therapy may represent over-treatment for some women with DCIS; this drug is associated not only with an increased risk of endometrial cancer but also thromboembolism. For patients with small low-grade lesions without comedonecrosis treatment with local excision alone may be adequate. Such patients have a low risk of relapse (3–4%) and any benefits from tamoxifen are likely to be modest and of the order 1–2%. By contrast, patients with larger, high-grade lesions will derive substantial benefit from tamoxifen when treated with local excision and radiotherapy rather than mastectomy (recurrence risk for ipsilateral breast cancer being 12% and 1%, respectively). The use of tamoxifen in conjunction with local excision and radiotherapy may avoid the need for mastectomy in those patients with localized DCIS but a relatively high Van Nuys score (7,8) whose risk of relapse at 10 years can be reduced to 5–10%[34].

Other Beneficial Effects of Tamoxifen

Several studies demonstrate that tamoxifen decreases total cholesterol and LDL levels in treated women[35]. However, serum triglycerides seem to increase and HDL levels remains unchanged. This beneficial effect on serum lipids reduces the risk of ischaemic heart disease. McDonald *et al.*[36] observed that the myocardial infarction (MI) rate was 14 per 1000 years at risk for the treatment group compared with 23 per 1000 for the control group. Tamoxifen has also been found to preserve or increase bone-mineral density in premenopausal and postmenopausal women treated with the drug[16].

Resistance to Tamoxifen

It is well recognized that almost all breast cancers that respond to tamoxifen with either tumour regression or disease stabilization eventually acquire resistance to this agent. It has been found that a high proportion of resistant tumours continue to express ER protein[37]. A percentage of these tamoxifen-resistant tumours which retain ER expression will respond to second-line endocrine therapy, although response rates will be less than for first-line therapies[38]. Multiple mechanisms appear to be implicated in development of tamoxifen resistance and include:

(a) Variations in co-regulatory proteins of the ER[39,40];
(b) Tamoxifen-stimulated growth resulting from emergence of clones of cells sensitive to the agonist properties of tamoxifen[41];
(c) Loss of and/or mutation of cellular receptors (mutations of the ER which include functionally active variants have been documented in breast cancer tissue, although their role remains uncertain)[42];
(d) Post-receptor mechanisms involving constitutive over-expression of mitogenic growth factors and their cognate receptors[43];
(e) ER-beta mediated mechanisms.

In recent years, interest has focussed on the role of co-regulatory proteins consisting of co-activators and co-repressors. Binding of these proteins determines the capacity of the tamoxifen–ER complex to influence oestrogen regulated gene transcription. For example, binding of co-repressors to the tamoxifen–ER complex would suppress the partial agonist activity of tamoxifen whereas co-activators would exert the opposite effect and enhance expression of oestrogen regulated genes. The conformational changes induced in the ER protein by tamoxifen determines the precise allosteric interactions with co-regulatory proteins which may represent a potential therapeutic target for novel therapies in patients with acquired tamoxifen resistance.

Tamoxifen and HER-2 Expression

HER-2 is a proto-oncogene that encodes a transmembrane tyrosine kinase receptor. There is an increasing body of evidence suggesting significant cross-talk between HER-2 receptor and ER. It has been hypothesized that HER-2 over-expression (25% of breast carcinoma) is associated with resistance to hormonal therapy. A recent metanalysis of HER-2 expression and response to hormonal therapy in women with metastatic breast cancer was presented at the ASCO meeting in New Orleans (May 2000). De Laurentiis and colleagues found that the overall odds ratio of disease progression was 2.46 (95% CI = 1.81–3.34) for HER-2 over-expressing tumours ($n = 1110$ patients)[44].

The complete data at 20 years of the Naples GUN randomized trial also indicated that tumours over-expressing HER-2 are unresponsive to tamoxifen[45]. However, caution should be exercised when interpreting results of studies that examine the role of HER-2 expression in predicting adjuvant tamoxifen failure because these are often retrospective studies which lack standardized methods of determining HER-2 status. Prospective trials using HER-2 status as a stratum for randomization are required.

Duration of Adjuvant Tamoxifen

The recent EBCTCG overview has confirmed that 5 years of adjuvant tamoxifen is of greater benefit than 2 years of therapy (EBCTCG 1998). An outstanding issue is whether tamoxifen treatment beyond 5 years confers additional benefits overall. This question is currently being addressed by the ATTom (Adjuvant Tamoxifen Treatment Offer More) and ATLAS (Adjuvant Tamoxifen – Longer Against Shorter) trials. The former recruits women with early breast cancer treated for 5 years with tamoxifen and no evidence of relapse. Patients are randomized to either continue tamoxifen for a further 5 years or to stop after the standard period of 5 years.

References

1. Colletta AA, Benson JR, Baum M. Alternate mechanisms of action of antioestrogens. *Breast Cancer Res Treat* 1994; **31**: 5–9.
2. Wakeling AE, Dukes M, Bowler J. A potent specific pure anti-oestrogen with clinical potential. *Cancer Res* 1991; **52**: 3867–3873.

3. Jordan VC. The development of tamoxifen for breast cancer therapy: a tribute to the late Arthur Walpole. *Breast Cancer Res Treat* 1988; **11**: 197–209.
4. Cole MP, Jones CTA, Todd IDH. A new antioestrogenic agent in breast cancer, a preliminary appraisal of ICI 46,474. *Br J Cancer* 1971; **25**: 270–275.
5. Ward HWC. Anti-oestrogen therapy for breast cancer: a trial of tamoxifen at low dose levels. *Br Med J* 1976; **1**: 13–15.
6. Nolvadex Adjuvant Trial Organisation. Controlled trial of tamoxifen as a single adjuvant agent in the management of early breast cancer. Interim analysis at four years. *Lancet* 1983; **1**, 257–261.
7. Nolvadex Adjuvant Trial Organisation. Controlled trial of tamoxifen as a single adjuvant agent in the management of early breast cancer. *Br J Cancer* 1988; **57**: 608–611.
8. Medical Research Council Scottish Trials Office. Adjuvant tamoxifen in the management of operable breast cancer. *Lancet* 1987; **11**: 171–175.
9. Fisher B, Constantino J, Redmond C *et al*. A randomized clinical trial evaluating tamoxifen in the treatment of patients with node negative breast cancer who have estrogen receptor negative tumours. *N Engl J Med* 1989; **320**: 479–484.
10. Colletta AA, Wakefield LM, Howell FV *et al*. Anti-oestrogens induce the secretion of active transforming growth factor beta from human foetal fibroblasts. *Br J Cancer* 1990; **62**: 405-409.
11. Potter GA, McCague R, Jarman M. A mechanistic hypothesis for DNA adduct formation by tamoxifen following hepatic oxidative metabolism. *Carcinogenesis* 1994; **15**: 439–442
12. Jordan VC, Glusman JE, Eckert S *et al*. Incident primary breast cancers are reduced by raloxifene: integrated data from multicenter, double blind, randomized trials in 12,000 post-menopausal women (abstract). *Proc Am Soc Clin Oncol* 1998; **17**: 122a.
13. Jordan CV. Tamoxifen for the treatment and prevention of breast cancer. *PRR* 1999; 257–263.
14. Fawell SE, Whiter, Hoare S *et al*. Inhibition of estrogen receptor-DNA binding by the pure anti-oestrogen ICI 164,384 appears to be mediated by impaired receptor dimerization. *Proc Natl Acad Sci (USA)* 1990; **87**: 6883–6887.
15. O' Brian CA, Liskamp RM, Solomon DH, Weinstein IB. Inhibition of protein kinase C by tamoxifen. *Cancer Res* 1985; **45**: 2462–2465.
16. Berridge MJ, Irving RF. Inositol triphosphate, a novel second messenger in cellular signal transduction. *Nature* 1984; **312**: 315–321.
17. O' Brian CA, Liskamp RM, Solomon DH, Weinstein IB. Triphenylethylenes: a new class of protein kinase C inhibitors. *J Natl Cancer Inst* 1986; **76**: 1243–1246.
18. Lam H-YP. Tamoxifen is a calmodulin antagonist in the activation of a cAMP phosphodiesterase. *Biochem Biophys Res Commun* 1984; **118**: 27–32.

19. Rowland MG, Parr IB, MacCague R *et al*. Variation of the inhibition of calmodulin dependent cyclic AMP phospho-diesterase among analogues of tamoxifen: correlation with cytotoxicity. *Biochem Pharmacol* 1990; **40**: 283–289.

20. Benson JR, Colletta AA Changes in expression of transforming growth factor beta mRNA isoforms in patients undergoing tamoxifen therapy (letter). *Br J Cancer* 1997; **75**: 776–778.

21. Butta A, Maclennan K, Flanders KC *et al*. Induction of transforming growth factor beta 1 in human breast cancer in vivo following tamoxifen treatment. *Cancer Res* 1992; **52**: 4261–4264.

22. Benson JR, LM Wakefield, MB Sporn *et al*. Synthesis and secretion of TGF-β isoforms by primary cultures of human breast tumour fibroblasts in vitro and their modulation by tamoxifen. *Br J Cancer* 1996; **74**: 352– 358.

23. Weidner N, Semple JP, Welch WR, Folkman J. Tumor angiogenesis and metastasis – correlation in invasive breast carcinoma. *N Engl J Med* 1991; **324**: 1–8.

24. Horak E, Harris AL. Angiogenesis, assessed by platelet/endothelial cell adhesion molecule antibodies, as indicator of node metastases and survival in breast cancer. *Lancet* 1992; **340**: 1120–1124.

25. Gagliardi A, Collins DC. Inhibition of angiogenesis by anti-estrogens. *Cancer Res* 1993; **53**: 533–535.

26. Heimark RL, Twardzik DR, Schwartz SM. Inhibition of endothelial regeneration by type-β transforming growth factor from platelets. *Science* 1986; **233**: 1078–1080.

27. Pollak M, Huynh HT, Pratt Lefebre S. Tamoxifen reduces serum insulin-like growth factor I (IGF I). *Breast Cancer Res Treat* 1992; **22**: 91–100.

28. Huynh HT, Tetenes E, Wallace L, Pollak M. *In vivo* inhibition of insulin-like growth factor I gene expression by tamoxifen. *Cancer Res* 1993; **53**: 1727– 1730.

29. Early Breast Cancer Trialists' Collaborative Group. Tamoxifen for early breast cancer. An overview of the randomised trials. *Lancet* 1998; **351**: 1451–1467.

30. Litherland S, Jackson IM. Antioestrogens in the management of hormone-dependent breast cancer. *Cancer Treat Rep* 1988; **15**: 183–194.

31. Williams MR, Todd JH, Ellis IO *et al*. Oestrogen receptors in primary and advanced breast cancer. An 8 year survival review of 704 cases. *Br J Cancer* 1987; **55**: 67–73.

32. Buchanan RB, Blamey RW, Durrant KR *et al*. A randomized comparison of tamoxifen with surgical oophorectomy in premenopausal patients with advanced breast cancer. *J Clin Oncol* 1986; **4**: 1326–1330.

33. Ravdin PM, Green S, Dorr TM *et al*. Prognostic significance of progesterone receptor levels in estrogen receptor-positive patients with metastatic breast cancer treated with tamoxifen. Results of a prospective Southwest Oncology Group study. *J Clin Oncol* 1992; **10**: 1284–1291.

34. Fisher B, Digname J, Wolmark N *et al.* Tamoxifen in treatment of intraductal breast cancer. National Surgical Adjuvant Breast and Bowel Project, B-24 randomised controlled trial. *Lancet* 1999; **353**: 1993–2000.
35. Bilimoria MM, Assikis VJ, Jordan VC. Should adjuvant tamoxifen therapy be stopped at 5 years? *Cancer J Sci Am* 1996; **2**: 140–150.
36. McDonald CC, Alexander FE, Whyte BW *et al.* Cardiac and vascular morbidity in women receiving adjuvant tamoxifen for breast cancer in a randomised trial. *Br Med J* 1995; **311**: 977–980.
37. Osborne CK. Tamoxifen in the treatment of breast cancer. *N Engl J Med* 1998; **339**: 1609–1618.
38. Howell A, Downey S, Anderson E. New endocrine therapies for breast cancer. *Eur J Cancer* 1996; **32A**: 576–588.
39. McKenna NJ, Lanz RB, O'Malley BW. Nuclear receptor corregulators cellular and molecular biology. *Endocr Rev* 1999; **20**: 321–344.
40. Norris JD, Paige LA, Christensen DJ *et al.* Peptide antagonists of the human estrogen receptor. *Science* 1999; **285**: 744–746.
41. Gottardis MM, Jordan VC. Development of tamoxifen-stimulated growth of MCF-7 tumours in athymic mice after long term antiestrogen stimulation. *Cancer Res* 1988; **48**: 5183–5187.
42. Fuqua SAW, Fitzgerald SD, Chamness G, Tandon AK, McDonnell DP. Variant human breast tumour oestrogen receptor with constitutive transcriptional activity. *Cancer Res* 1991; **51**: 105–109
43. LeRoy X, Escot C, Brouillet JP, Theillet C, Maudelonde T, Simony-Lafontaine J, Pujol H, Rochefort H. Decrease of cerbB2 and c-myc RNA levels in tamoxifen treated breast cancer. *Oncogene* 1991; **6**: 431–437
44. De Laurentiis M, Arpino G, Massarelli E *et al.* A metanalysis of the interaction between Her2 and the response to endocrine therapy in metastatic breast cancer. *Proc Am Soc Clin Oncol* 2000; **78a**: Abstr 300.
45. Bianco AR, De Laurentiis M, Carlomagno C *et al.* Her2 overexpression predicts adjuvant tamoxifen failure for early breast cancer: complete data at 20 years of the Naples GUN randomized trial. *Proc Am Soc Clin Oncol* 2000; **75**: Abstr 289.

5. Raloxifene

J. C. C. Hu and K. Mokbel

Introduction

The discovery that the antiestrogen tamoxifen was not purely an antagonist of the estrogen receptors (ERs) and it was a drug that bound with strong affinity to the receptor ERs but could act as antagonist on some tissues but as agonists on others, led to the development of the concept of selective estrogen receptor modulators (SERMs). This notion inspired vigorous research into the development of an ideal SERM which would be effective in the prevention and treatment of breast cancer, osteoporosis, ischaemic heart disease and Alzheimer's disease without increasing the risk of endometrial cancer and venous thromboembolism or the side-effects of conventional hormone replacement therapy (HRT). Raloxifene (Evista) is a SERM which meets many of the 'ideal' criteria and many randomized controlled trials evaluating the drug are underway.

History

The first non-steroidal antiestrogen was discovered in 1958 by Lerner and co-workers. The estrogen receptor which was identified in 1960 by Jensen and Jacobsen provided a target for drug action. Tamoxifen, the first antiestrogen, now classified to be SERM, initially used in the treatment of breast cancer, has been recently used for prevention. In addition, it seems to have an estrogenic affect on bone and results in a decreased incidence of osteoporosis. This caused a paradigm shift which resulted in the development of a drug which could prevent osteoporosis with the beneficial side-effect of preventing breast cancer[1]. With this concept, in the 1980s, raloxifene (Evista) was developed by Lilly. Since then, many trials have been set up to assess the benefits and risks of the drug.

Mechanism of Action

Raloxifene hydrochloride is a non-steroidal benzothiopene. It binds to ER with a high affinity and has antiestrogenic effects in breast and uterus but estrogenic effects in bone and liver. The mechanism of action of raloxifene has not been elucidated completely but there are a couple of postulates.

By using protein crystallography, it has been demonstrated that when raloxifene binds to an estrogen receptor, a conformational change occurs which is different from that following the binding of estrogen to the same receptor[2]. Furthermore, it is likely that within the class of SERMs each drug causes slightly different conformational changes. It could be these subtle differences that result in the different drug profiles. Raloxifene may be also acting through a different isoform of ER rather than ER-alpha. ER-beta has been discovered recently, but the relationship is not clear.

Raloxifene and Osteoporosis

As a drug developed primarily for osteoporosis in 1996, a multicentre randomized study called the Multiple Outcome of Raloxifene Evaluation (MORE) trial was set up. This study, which is still ongoing, enrolled 7705 women who were postmenopausal, under 80 years of age, and had osteoporosis defined as spine fracture and/or hip spine bone density at least 2.5 standard deviations below normal for young Caucasian women. They were randomized to placebo, 60 mg/day or 120 mg/day of raloxifene and they all received calcium and vitamin D supplements. The selection criteria were extremely stringent – some of the relevant exclusion criteria, for example, were women with prior breast or endometrial cancer and abnormal uterine bleeding. The primary endpoint was to assess whether raloxifene could reduce vertebral fractures. Other fractures such as wrist and pelvis were also included as secondary endpoints.

The initial results at 3 years of follow-up indicated that bone density was increased by an average of 2.35% at the dose of 60 mg/day and 2.55% at the dose of 120 mg/day at the femoral neck and lumbar spine respectively. These beneficial effects were over and above improvements seen with the intake of dietary calcium and vitamin D. Also, a substantial decrease in bone turnover markers such as osteocalcin and type 1 collagen C-telopeptide by 33% was observed[3]. The relative risk of vertebral fracture was 0.7 and 0.5 for the doses of 60 mg/day and 120 mg/day of raloxifene respectively. The reduction in fractures was greater than expected from the modest improvement in bone density. However, the risk of non-vertebral fracture did not differ significantly between placebo and raloxifene groups[4]. Unlike tamoxifen[5], raloxifene has not been found to reduce the risk of non-vertebral fractures. However, longer follow-up is required to address this end-point.

Raloxifene and Breast Cancer

It is generally accepted that there is a strong association between endogenous estrogen and the subsequent development of breast cancer. Tamoxifen, a SERM with antiestrogenic effects in the breast, has been used for both treatment and prevention with good results. However, there are worrying side-effects such as endometrial cancer[6], retinopathy and menopausal symptoms. Raloxifene, although primarily developed for osteoporosis, because of its estrogen antagonist activity in the breast, may have the spin-off benefit of treating or preventing breast cancer. There have been no trials in using raloxifene to treat breast cancer. This may be because tamoxifen is an extremely effective treatment and there is a vast amount of literature and experience in using it.

Raloxifene has been proposed for use as a chemopreventative agent. The advantage over tamoxifen is that it does not stimulate the endometrium and does not increase the risk of cancer. As a secondary end-point of the MORE trial, it has been found that at both 60 mg and 120 mg doses of raloxifene, there is a 90% reduction in the risk of developing ER-positive tumour. Not surprisingly there is no apparent effect on the risk of developing ER-negative tumour. Overall the risk of development of breast cancer was reduced by 76%[7]. Therefore it is questionable whether the drug would be useful in preventing genetic cancers as most BRCA 1-positive women develop ER-negative tumours. As the effect of raloxifene on breast cancer risk was examined as a secondary endpoint, the multiplicity issue remains a source of bias in this study.

Therefore there is need to validate these results by randomized controlled trial with reducing the risk of development of breast cancer as a primary endpoint. The study of tamoxifen and raloxifene (STAR), underway in the USA and Canada, plans to recruit 22 000 high-risk postmenopausal women into the trial. They are randomized to tamoxifen 20 mg or raloxifene 60 mg daily. The ultimate aim is to evaluate breast cancer incidence at 7 years and whether one drug is superior to the other. Cauley *et al.* have recently presented an update of the MORE study with 48 months of follow-up and confirmed the chemo-preventative effect of raloxifene[8].

Nevertheless there are still many questions to be answered. For example, the length of time that the drug has to be taken to obtain the maximum benefit, whether the protective effect lasts after cessation of the drug and, if so, the length of time and which subgroup of patients would benefit the most.

Raloxifene and Hormone Replacement Therapy (HRT)

With its estrogenic effect in bone and its antiestrogenic effects in breast and endometrium, raloxifene has been proposed for use as an alternative to HRT. However, it does not relieve several menopausal symptoms such as hot flushes (a common side-effect of raloxifene), vaginal dryness or urethritis. Such symptoms are still best treated with HRT. It is easy to see that it is extremely tempting to use this drug in postmenopausal women who have minimal menopausal symptoms and have no history of deep vein thrombosis but who are at risk from osteoporosis and breast cancer. It is unlikely, however, that raloxifene will replace HRT entirely as it does not combat important postmenopausal symptoms. Whether raloxifene will be most beneficial to a subgroup of postmenopausal women remains to be determined in suitable clinical trials.

Raloxifene and the Endometrium

The major concern in using tamoxifen in the prevention and treatment of breast cancer is its estrogenic effects on the endometrium and the subsequent increase in the risk of endometrial cancer[6]. Several randomized controlled trials[9,10] have shown that there is no stimulatory effect on the endometrium. As mentioned earlier, this is a significant advantage of the drug.

Raloxifene and Cardiovascular Disease

Heart disease is a major killer in the Western world and estrogen has been thought to be cardioprotective, as the incidence of heart disease rises exponentially in postmenopausal women. It has been found that HRT reduces LDL cholesterol and raises HDL cholesterol. The overall risk of developing heart disease seems to be lower for women taking HRT. The Heart and Estrogen/Progestin Replacement Study (HERS)[12] found no cardioprotective effect with estrogen and medroxy-progesterone acetate. The first large clinical trial involved 2763 women with an average age of 67 years and had confirmed coronary heart disease. They were randomized to either placebo or combined HRT.

The effect of raloxifene on the cardiovascular system has also been intensely investigated. Its potential cardioprotective effect was initially discovered in animal studies. There was a decrease in serum cholesterol in ovariectomized rats[12] and limited cholesterol accumulation in the aorta of ovariectomized, cholesterol-fed rabbits[13] after the intake of raloxifene. As a secondary finding, the MORE trial also found that raloxifene reduced LDL cholesterol but had no effect on HDL cholesterol and also lowered the level of lipoprotein and fibrinogen. However, whether these changes translate into better outcome clinically is still unknown. A large case controlled trial, Raloxifen Use for the Heart (RUTH) trial due to be complete in 2005, has been set up to assess whether raloxifene prevents heart disease by looking at endpoints such as myocardial infarction and coronary deaths. The plan is to recruit 10 000 postmenopausal women over 55 years of age either with, or at high risk, of coronary artery disease. This trial hopefully will give the answer as to whether raloxifene can be used as an agent to prevent cardiovascular disease.

Side-effects

Table 1 Percentage rates of side-effects in the MORE trial. Adapted from Cummings et al.[6]

Adverse effects	Placebo	Raloxifene 60 mg/day	Raloxifene 120 mg/day
Thromboembolic disease	0.3	1.0	0.8
Hot flushes	6.4	9.7	11.6
Leg cramps	3.7	7.0	6.9
Peripheral oedema	4.4	5.2	6.5
Diabetes mellitus	0.5	1.2	1.1

Apart from the beneficial effects of raloxifene, there are also side-effects. The most important side-effects are the increased risk of venous thromboembolism. It is three times higher in patients taking raloxifene but does not seem to be dose related[6]. Therefore, the drug should not be used in patients with a previous history of DVTs. Other less dangerous side-effects include hot flushes, leg cramps, peripheral oedema and diabetes mellitus. Overall, the pros of raloxifene seem to outweigh the cons.

Other SERMs

Toremifene is a chlorotamoxifen that has been recently marketed for breast cancer. A recent study of the three doses of toremifene has shown that 40 and 60 mg daily are effective and safe in postmenopausal women with advanced breast cancer[14]. The safety and efficacy results of a randomized trial comparing adjuvant toremifene (40 mg daily) and tamoxifen (20 mg daily) in postmenopausal women with node-positive breast cancer have recently been reported[15]. The authors observed that the efficacy and safety profiles of toremifene were similar to that of tamoxifen. LY353381 is a new SERM with strong breast antiestrogen and negligible agonist activity on the uterus. A recent phase II trial of two doses of LY353381 (20 and 50 mg daily) in metastatic and locally-advanced breast cancer has demonstrated efficacy and safety. Phase III trials are currently being planned. Several other SERMs such as idoxifene, droloxifene, nafoxidene, zindoxifene, ZK119010, LY156758, LY117018 and benzopyrans are currently in clinical development. All these drugs are non-steroidal and have antiestrogenic and partial agonist activity.

Conclusions

Raloxifene is an extremely exciting drug with multifunctional activity. By understanding the mechanism of SERMs, it may be possible to develop an 'ideal' drug without the side-effects. Raloxene is an established drug for both prevention and treatment of osteoporosis. As more data are accrued, it is likely that it will be an effective drug in the prevention of breast cancer and perhaps treatment. The purported usage as a preventative drug for cardiovascular disease is unsubstantiated at present. However, randomized controlled trial will provide further information. It seems that raloxifene may benefit a small subgroup of postmenopausal women as an HRT. Again, this concept needs to be investigated further.

References

1. Lerner LJ, Jordan VC. Development of antiestrogens and their use in breast cancer. *Cancer Res* 1990; **50**: 4177–4189.
2. Brzozowski AM, Pike ACW, Dauter Z *et al.* Molecular basis of agonism in the oestrogen receptor. *Nature* 1997; **389**: 753–758.
3. Ettinger B, Black DM, Miltak BH *et al.* Reduction of vertebral fracture in post menopausal women with osteoporosis treated with raloxifene: results from a 3 year randomised clinical trial. Multiple Outcomes of Raloxifene Evaluation (MORE) Investigators. *JAMA* 1999; **282**: 637–645.
4. Fisher B, Constantino JP, Wickerham DL *et al.* Tamoxifen for prevention of breast cancer: report of the National Surgical Adjuvant Breast and Bowel Project P-1 study. *J Nat Cancer Inst* 1998; **90**: 1371–1381.
5. Dijkhuizen FPHIJ, Brolmann HAM, Oddens BJJ *et al.* Transvaginal ultrasonography and endometrial changes in postmenopausal breast cancer patients receiving tamoxifen. *Maturitas* 1996; **25**: 45–50.
6. Cummings SR, Eckert S, Kreuger KA *et al.* The effect of raloxifene on the risk of breast cancer in postmenopausal women: results from the MORE randomised trial. *JAMA* 1999; **281**: 2189–2197.
7. Cauley J, Kruegger K, Eckert S *et al.* Breast cancer risk in postmenopausal women with osteoporosis is reduced with raloxifene treatment: extension

of the MORE trial data to a median follow-up of 48 months. *Proc Am Soc Clin Oncol* 2000; **88a**: Abstr. 356.

8. Delmas PD, Bajarnson NH, Mitlak BH *et al*. Effects of raloxifene on bone mineral density, serum cholesterol concentrations and uterine endometrium in postmenopausal women. *N Engl J Med* 1997; **337**: 1641–1647.

9. Goldstein S, Srikanth R, Parsons A *et al*. Effects of raloxifene on the endometrium in healthy postmenopausal women. *Menopause* 1998; **5**: 277.

10. Barrett-Conor E, Grady D, Hormone replacement therapy, heart disease and other considerations. *Annu Rev Public Health* 1998; **19**: 55–57.

11. Hulley S, Grady D, Bush T *et al*. Randomised trial of estrogen plus progestin for secondary prevention of coronary heart disease in post-menopausal women. Heart and Estrogen/Progestin Replacement Study (HERS) Research Group. *JAMA* 1998; **280**: 605–613.

12. Bjarnson NH, Haarbo J, Byrjalsen I *et al*. Raloxifene inhibits aortic accumulation of cholesterol in ovariectomised cholesterol fed rabbits. *Circulation* 1997; **96**: 1964–1969.

13. Ellmen J, Hakulinen P, Edwards M *et al*. Hormonal effects of three toremifene (Fareston) doses in postmenopausal women with breast cancer. *Proc Am Soc Clin Oncol* 2000; **19**: 102a.

14. Holli K, Valavaara R, Blanco G, *et al*. Safety and efficacy results of a randomised trial comparing adjuvant toremifene and tamoxifen in postmenopausal patients with node-positive breast cancer. *J Clin Oncol* 2000; **18**: 3487–3494.

6. Anti-aromatase Agents

K. Mokbel

Introduction

Estrogens play an important role in the development and growth of hormone-dependent breast tumours[1,2]. The main sites of estrogen biosynthesis in postmenopausal women are skin, muscle, adipose tissue and benign and malignant breast tissue[3–5]. In such tissues, estrogen (C_{18} steroid) is derived from androgens (C_{19} steroids) by the aromatase complex. This group of drugs inhibits the cytochrome P-450 component of the aromatase enzyme by interfering with the electron transfer from NADPH. Anastrozole (Arimidex) and letrozole (Femara) are examples of such agents. Aromatase inhibitors can be also classified into first-generation (e.g. aminoglutethimide), second-generation (e.g. formestane and fadrazole) and third-generation (e.g. anastrozole, letrozole and exemestane) compounds. Two types of drug can inhibit aromatase. The type I inhibitors have a steroidal structure similar to androgens and inactivate the enzyme irreversibility by blocking the substrate-binding site and are therefore known as aromatase inactivators. Examples of such drugs include formestane and exemestane (Aromasin). Type II inhibitors are non-steroidal and their action is reversible. The conversion of adrenal androstenedione to estrone by aromatase is related to body weight[6]. In normal weight subjects, approximately 1% of androstenedione is converted to estrone whereas in obese subjects, this increases up to 10%. The increase in peripheral estrogen synthesis with weight in postmenopausal women is the most likely explanation for the increased risk of breast cancer observed in obese postmenopausal women[6]. Aromatase activity seems also to increase with ageing[7]. Figure 1 demonstrates the structure of important aromatase inhibitors.

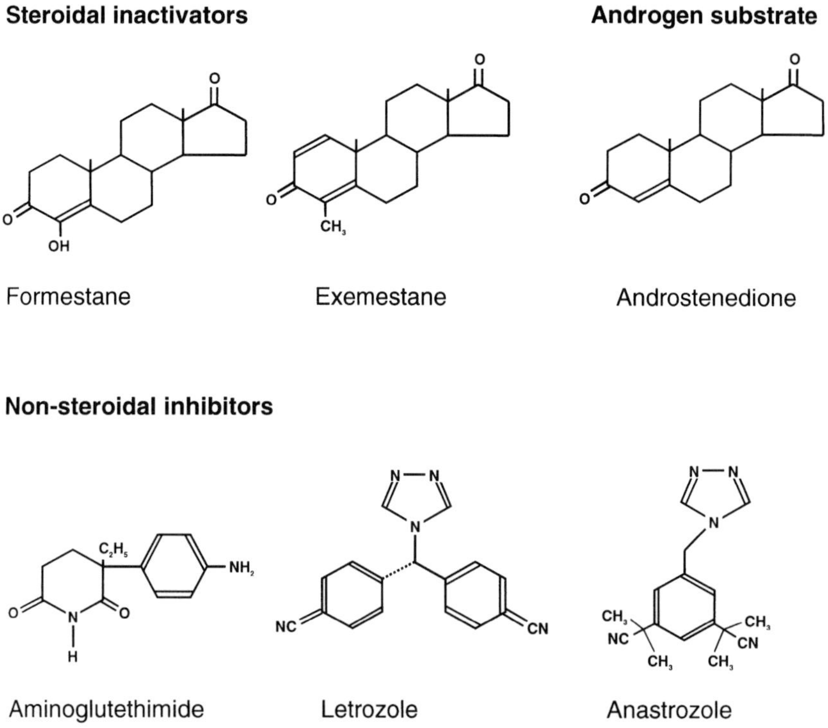
Steroidal inactivators
Androgen substrate
O
OH
CH3
Formestane
Exemestane
Androstenedione
Non-steroidal inhibitors
C2H5
NH2
N
H
NC
CN
N—N
N
CH3
Aminoglutethimide
Letrozole
Anastrozole

Figure 1 Structure of aromatase inhibitors

Anastrozole (Arimidex)

Two international phase III randomized trials have been conducted to compare the efficacy and tolerability of anastrozole with that of megestrol acetate (Megace) in postmenopausal women who had relapsed/recurred on adjuvant tamoxifen treatment or following tamoxifen therapy for advanced breast cancer[8]. However, the publications represent a combined analysis of two independently-conducted trials of the same protocol design with few details of the results of the individual trials. One study was carried out in Europe, Australia and South Africa and included 378 patients; the other study involved 386 patients from the USA and Canada. All patients had evaluable disease and 70% of them had ER-positive tumours. The remainder were ER-negative (5%) or of unknown ER status (25%). The patients were randomized into three areas: anastrozole 1 mg o.d., anastrozole 10 mg once daily (o.d.) and megestrol acetate 40 mg q.d.s. Both studies were double-blinded to anastrozole dose only but not to megestrol acetate. The end points of the trials included objective response rate (CR and PR), time to tumour progression (TTP), time to treatment failure (TTF), duration of response, survival and tolerability. The UICC criteria and computerized algorithms based on tumour measurements were used to assess response. Clinical benefit analyses were conducted after median follow-up period of 6 and 31 months. Tolerability data were assessed at median follow-up period of 6 and 12 months. The 6-month analysis revealed that both doses of anastrozole were as effective as megestrol acetate in terms of overall clinical benefit and time to disease progression. The 10 mg dose had no additional clinical benefit over the 1 mg dose, therefore it was decided that the 1 mg dose would be used after tamoxifen failure. At 31 months, the data were mature enough to allow survival analysis. The 2-year survival was 56.1% for the anastrozole group compared with 46.3% for the Megace group (hazard ratio = 0.78, 97.5% CI = 0.6040–0.9996, $p = 0.0248$). The median survival was 26.7 months and 22.5 months for patients receiving Arimidex and Megace respectively. The survival benefit was not statistically significant in the North American study. There were no significant differences between the two treatments in terms of objective response (CR and PR) and stable disease (SD) ≥ 24 weeks. The duration of overall clinical benefit for anastrozole was 18.3 months. Tolerability data showed that Arimidex was generally well tolerated with less weight gain ($p < 0.01$) than Megace and less than 3% of patients withdrawing from the treatment due to unacceptable side-effects. Quality of life data was not reported in these studies. Arimidex is currently being used widely as a second line therapy in postmenopausal women who relapse on (or fail to respond to tamoxifen therapy). The contraindications to Arimidex use include severe renal impairment (creatinine clearance <20 ml/min), severe hepatic impairment, premenopausal patients and concomitant use of estrogens.

A recent combined analysis of two identically designed multicentre trials has demonstrated that anastrozole was superior to tamoxifen in prolonging time to tumour progression (TTP) in postmenopausal women with advanced breast cancer (ER positive and/or PgR positive). Furthermore there were fewer side-effects (thromboembolic events and vaginal bleeding) in the anastrozole arm. Such data suggest that anastrazole could be used as an alternative to tamoxifen in postmenopausal women with hormonally-sensitive advanced breast cancer[9].

Letrozole (Femara)

Two randomized multicentre trials compared letrozole with megestrol acetate[10] (160 mg o.d.) and aminoglutethimide[11] (250 mg q.d.s). Two doses of letrozole (2.5 mg and 0.5 mg o.d.) were used in the treatment group. All patients had measurable/evaluable disease at trial entry. In the letrozole versus megestrol acetate study, 544 patients were randomized to three treatment arms. Letrozole 0.5 mg o.d., letrozole 2.5 mg o.d. and Megace 160 mg o.d. The study was double-blinded unlike that of anastrozole versus Megace and had the combined response rate (RR) as its primary end point. The latter was defined as RR = CR + PR. The UICC criteria for assessing response were used. A total of 57% of patients were ER positive. Data analysis showed that letrozole was superior to megestrol acetate in terms of RR (24 vs 16%, $p = 0.04$), duration of response ($p = 0.01$), TTP (5.6 vs 5.5 months, $p = 0.07$), TTF (5.1 vs 3.9 months, $p = 0.04$), tolerability and quality of life. However, there was no significant difference in the overall survival (25 vs 22 months, $p = 0.15$). When compared with aminoglutethimide, letrozole was found to be superior in terms of RR (20 vs 12% NS), duration of response (34 vs 15 months, NS) TTP ($p = 0.004$), TTF ($p = 0.001$), overall survival ($p = 0.002$) and toxicity ($p > 0.05$). This trial did not report quality of life data. In both studies, the dose of 2.5 mg was found to be superior to 0.5 mg. Despite exercising caution when making indirect comparisons between letrozole and anastrozole, it is reasonable to postulate/speculate that the *in vivo* superiority of letrozole in aromatase inhibition[12] may explain the observation that letrozole, but not anastrozole, was more efficacious than Megace. Mouridsen and colleagues[13] have recently presented the results of a phase III clinical trial comparing letrozole with tamoxifen as a first-line therapy in postmenopausal women with locally-advanced or metastatic breast cancer ($n = 907$) The median TTP was significantly longer in patients taking letrozole (2.5 mg once daily) compared with those taking tamoxifen (41 and 26 weeks respectively, $p = 0.0001$). Such results suggest that letrozole should be used as a first-line therapy in postmenopausal women with advanced breast cancer (ER and/or PgR positive) in preference to tamoxifen. Although the data suggest that letrozole may be superior to anastrazole in this setting (median TTP = 41 and 34 weeks respectively), caution should be exercised when making indirect comparison and this question is best answered by randomized controlled trials comparing the two drugs head to head. Ellis *et al.*[14] have recently reported the results of a randomized double-blind multicentre trial comparing letrozole and tamoxifen in postmenopausal patients (n = 337) with ER- and/or PgR-positive tumours larger than 2 cm which were unsuitable for breast conserving surgery (BCS). The authors observed that preoperative letrozole for 4 months had a significantly higher objective response rate than tamoxifen (55% and 36% respectively, $p < 0.001$). Furthermore, the rate of BCS was significantly higher in the letrozole group (45% versus 35% respectively, $p = 0.022$). Therefore postmenopausal women with hormone receptor positive tumours unsuitable for BCS should be considered for neoadjuvant letrozole therapy.

Vorozole (Rivizor)

Two randomized multicentre trials compared Vorozole with megestrol acetate[15] and aminoglutethimide[16]. Neither study was blinded. The vorozole (2.5 mg o.d.) versus megestrol acetate (40 mg q.d.s) trial involved 432 women from 66 centres. The percentage of patients with ER-positive tumours was higher than the trials of anastrozole and letrozole. There as no statistically significant benefit over Megace in terms of combined response rate ($p = 0.29$), duration of response ($p = 0.20$), TTP (2.7 vs 3.6 months, $p = 0.46$) or overall survival (26 vs 29 months, $p = 0.93$). However, vorozole was significantly superior to Megace in terms of toxicity and weight gain. This trial design was thought to introduce bias by its schedule of response evaluations. The organs that were not involved at entry were not required systemically to be followed up. This was heavily criticized by the American Food and Drug Administration (FDA) and led to the suspension of registration procedures. The vorozole versus aminoglutethimide study involved 556 postmenopausal women (51% ER positive) from 74 centres. Vorozole was found to be superior in terms of combined response rate (23 vs 18%, $p = 0.07$), TTF (5.3 vs 4.4 months, $p = 0.04$), quality of life ($p = 0.014$) and toxicity ($p < 0.001$). There was no significant difference with respect to duration of response and TTP in contrast to the vorozole vs megestrol trial, the malignant disease was measurable or evaluable in this study.

Exemestane (Aromasin)

This is a new steroid, irreversible aromatase inactivator which has been developed for the palliative and adjuvant therapy of breast cancer. In a phase III randomized, multicentre, double-blinded study exemestane (25 mg/day) was compared with megestrol acetate (40 mg q.d.s) in 769 postmenopausal women with advanced breast cancer which had become refractory to tamoxifen therapy[17]. There was no significant difference between the two groups (366 vs 403) in baseline characteristics nor prognostic factors: performance status, sites of disease, hormonal receptor status and measurable disease (78% in both groups). Exemestane was significantly better than MA in terms of median time to progression (4.7 vs 3.8 months) duration of overall success (13.8 vs 11.3 months) and overall survival (Figure 2). The median survival was 28.4 months for MA but has not been reached yet with Aromasin. Furthermore, the study showed that exemestane was better tolerated than MA with a withdrawal rate of 1.4% (vs 2.5% with MA). The commonest reported side-effects were hot flushes (6%), nausea (9.2%) and fatigue (7.5%). The number of patients gaining weight was significantly lower in the exemestane arm (7.6 vs 5.1%, $p = 0.001$). Exemestane was also found to be effective as a third line therapy after failure of other third-generation aromatase inhibitors in approximately 25% of cases. Furthermore, exemestane caused profound suppression (= 90%) of estradiol, estrone and estrone sulphate levels in the serum. This suppression was maintained over time.

Subgroup analysis has also demonstrated a significantly higher objective response rates for lung and liver metastases with exemestane compared with MA. In contrast, no survival advantage has been reported in the clinical trials comparing of letrozole with MA[10,11]. In the clinical trials comparing anastrozole with MA, the median duration of objective response and overall success at the median time to treatment failure were not reported. However, the authors observed a survival advantage for anastrozole over MA in the combined analysis of the mature data of both arms of the study (North American and European arms) but not in the North American arm of the study[9].

Parideans *et al.* have recently presented the results of a phase II trial comparing exemestane (Aromasin) with tamoxifen in 97 postmenopausal women with metastatic breast cancer[18]. Data were available on 63 patients and showed that exemestane was well tolerated and effective as a first line therapy in postmenopausal women with metastatic disease. The authors have already commenced a phase III trial the results of which will be available within the next 2 years.

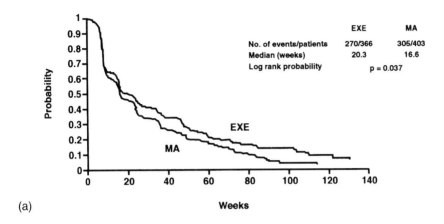

(a)

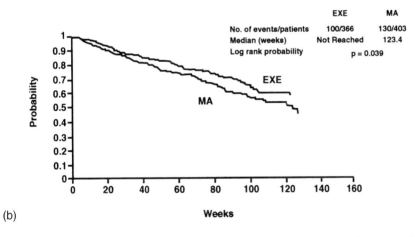

(b)

Figure 2 Kaplan–Meier curves for (a) time to tumour progression and (b) survival in postmenopausal women (*n* = 769) with advanced breast cancer randomized to exemestane (EXE) or megestrol acetate (MA). Adapted from Kaufmann *et al. J Clin Oncol* 2000; 18: 1399–1411

Conclusions

The new non-steroidal and steroidal aromatase inhibitors are at least as effective as megestrol acetate as second line hormonal agents in postmenopausal women with breast cancer. However, they are superior to MA in terms of tolerability and adverse effects. Letrozole and exemestane have been shown to be superior to MA in terms of efficacy. Furthermore, exemestane and anastrozole demonstrated a survival advantage over MA. There is a growing body of evidence supporting the role of third-generation aromatase inhibitors as first-line therapy for ER and/or PgR-positive advanced breast cancer in posmenopausal women, and as a neoadjuvant therapy in postmenopausal women with hormone receptor positive tumours unsuitable for breast conserving surgery. Boccardo *et al.*[19] have recently reported that the sequential use of adjuvant tamoxifen for 3 years followed by aminoglutethimide for 2 years does not seem to impact on disease recurrence compared with tamoxifen for 5 years. However, the sequential treatment has been associated with higher overall survival ($p = 0.006$). Such results suggest that third-generation aromatase inhibitors are very likely to be effective in the adjuvant setting. Studies comparing these drugs head-to-head and with tamoxifen are currently in progress. The potential role of these drugs in breast cancer prevention is worth investigating.

References

1. James VHT, Reed MJ. Steroid hormones and human cancer. *Prog Cancer Res Ther* 1980; **14**: 471–487.
2. Bernstein L, Ross RK. Endogenous hormones and breast cancer risk. *Epidemiol Rev* 1993; **15**: 48–65.
3. Siiteri PK, MacDonald PC. Role of extraglandular estrogen in human endocrinology. In Greep RO Astwood EB, eds, *Handbook of Physiology*. Washington DC: American Physiological Society, 1973; **2**: 615–629.
4. Reed MJ, Hutton JD, Baxendale PM *et al.* The conversion of androstenedione to oestrone and production of oestrone in women with endometrial cancer. *J Steroid Biochem* 1979; **11**: 905–911.
5. Grodin JM, Siiteri PK, MacDonald PC. Source of estrogen production in postmenopausal women. *J Clin Endocrinol Metab* 1973; **36**: 207–214.
6. Dunn LJ, Bradbury JT. Endocrine factors in endometrial carcinoma: a preliminary report. *Am J Obstet Gynecol* 1967; **97**: 465–471.

7.   Hemsell DL, Grodin JM, Brenner PF *et al.* Plasma precursors of estrogen. II. Correlation of the extent of conversion of plasma androstenedione to estrone with age. *J Clin Endocrin Metab* 1974; **38**: 476–479.

8.   Buzdar AU, Jonat W, Howell A *et al.* Anastrozole versus megestrol acetate in the treatment of postmenopausal women with advanced breast carcinoma: results of a survival update based on a combined analysis of data from two mature phase III trials. Arimidex Study Group. *Cancer* 1998; **83**: 1142–1152.

9.   Buzdar A, Nabholtz JM, Robertson JF *et al.* Anastrozole versus tamoxifen as first-line therapy for advanced breast cancer in postmenopausal women: Combined analysis from two identically designed multicentre trials. *Proc Am Soc Clin Oncol* 2000; **154a**: Abstr 609D.

10. Dombernowsky P, Smith I, Falkson G *et al.* Letrozole, a new oral aromatase inhibitor for advanced breast cancer: double-blind randomised trial showing a dose effect and improved efficacy and tolerability compared with megestrol acetate. *J Clin Oncol* 1998; **18**: 453–461.

11. Gershanovich M, Chaudhuri HA, Campos D *et al.* Letrozole, a new oral aromatase inhibitor: randomised trial comparing 2.5 mg daily, 0.5 mg daily and aminoglutethimide in postmenopausal women with advanced breast cancer. *Ann Oncol* 1998; **9**: 639–645.

12. Dowsett M, Geisler J, Haynes BP, *et al.* Letrozole achieves more complete inhibition of whole body aromatisation than anastrazole. *Eur J Cancer* 2000; **36**: S88–S89.

13. Mouridsen H, Pérez-Carrión R, Becquart D, *et al.* Letrozole (Femara) versus tamoxifen: preliminary data of a first-line clinical trial in postmenopausal women with locally advanced or metastatic breast cancer. *Eur J Cancer* 2000; **36**: S88.

14. Ellis MJ, Jaenicke F, Llombart-Cussac A, *et al.* A randomized double-blind multicentre study of preoperative tamoxifen versus Femara (letrozole) for postmenopausal women with ER and/or PgR positive breast cancer ineligible for breast conserving surgery – correlation of clinical response with tumour gene expression and proliferation. *Breast Cancer Res Treat* 2000; **64**: 29.

15. Gross P, Winer E, Tannock I *et al.* Vorozol vs Megace in postmenopausal patients with metastatic breast carcinoma who had relapsed following tamoxifen. *J Clin Oncol* 1997; **16**: 155a (Abstr. 542).

16. Bengtsson NO, Focan C, Gudgeon A *et al.* A phase III trial comparing Vorozole (Rivizor™) versus aminoglutethimide in the treatment of advanced postmenopausal breast cancer. *Eur J Cancer* 1997; **33**: S148 (Abstr. 656).

17. Kaufmann M, Bajeta E, Dirix LY *et al.* Exemestane is superior to megestrol acetate after tamoxifen failure in postmenopausal women with advanced breast cancer: results of a phase III randomised double blind trials. *J Clin Oncol* 2000; **18**: 1399–1411.

18. Paridaens R, Dirix LY, Beex L *et al.* Exemestane (Aromasin) is active and well tolerated as first line hormonal therapy of metastatic breast cancer

patients: results of a randomized phase II trial. *Proc Am Soc Clin Oncol* 2000; **83a**: Abstr. 316.

19. Boccardo F, Rubagotti A, Amoroso D *et al*. Tamoxifen vs amino-glutethimide in breast cancer patients previously treated with adjuvant tamoxifen. Preliminary results of a multicentric comparative study. *Proc Am Soc Clin Oncol* 2000; **71a**: Abstr. 273.

7. Pure Antiestrogens

K. Mokbel

Fulvestrant (Faslodex)

Introduction

The complex molecular biology of the estrogen receptor (ER) and the evidence that estrogen promotes the development and growth of breast cancer have led to the development of a new class of drugs that block the ER with no agonist activity. This feature differentiates these pure antiestrogens from SERMs such as tamoxifen and raloxifene which have agonist effects in certain tissues such as bone, serum lipids, liver and endometrium. Faslodex (ICI 182 780) is an important example of such pure antagonists.

Faslodex is a 7α-alkylsulfinyl analogue of estradiol (Figure 1) that lacks agonist activity. The relative affinity for the ER is 0.9 compared with estradiol. The drug also down-regulates ER and is therefore known as a selective estrogen receptor down-regulator (SERD).

Mechanism of Action

Faslodex inhibits transcription induced by all three transcriptional activating domains of the estrogen receptor. Furthermore, it enhances the degradation of ER thus optimizing hormonal therapy (Figure 2). Other mechanisms of action that may contribute to its antitumour activity include antiprogestin effects[1] and down-regulation of IGF-I[2].

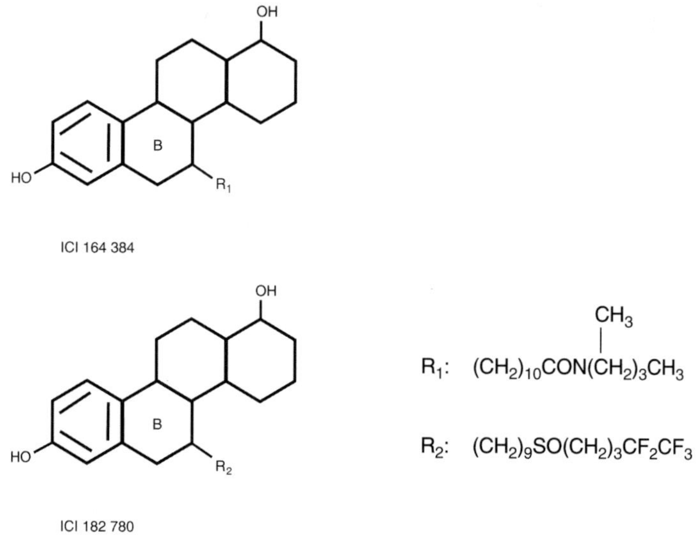

OH

B

HO

R$_1$

ICI 164 384

OH

B

HO

R$_2$

ICI 182 780

$$R_1: \quad (CH_2)_{10}CON(CH_2)_3CH_3$$
with CH$_3$ branch

$$R_2: \quad (CH_2)_9SO(CH_2)_3CF_2CF_3$$

Figure 1 Structure of pure antiestrogens ICI 164 384 and ICI 182 780. The 17β-estradiol structure is identical to ICI 164 384 and ICI 182 780 (Faslodex) except that it lacks side-chains R$_1$ and R$_2$ at the 7α position of the B ring

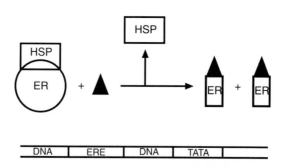

| DNA | ERE | DNA | TATA |

Figure 2 Mechanism of action of pure antiestrogens ICI 164 384 and ICI 182 780 (Faslodex) (▲). The binding of Faslodex to ER prevents dimerization and therefore no interaction between ER and ERE occurs

Pre-Clinical Studies

The *in vitro* growth inhibitory potency of Faslodex exceeded that of tamoxifen in ER-positive MCF-7 human breast cancer cell lines with greater reduction of the proportion of cells engaged in DNA synthesis in Faslodex-treated cells[3]. The binding affinity of Faslodex for ER is 100 times greater than that of tamoxifen in rats. The *in vivo* growth-inhibitory effects were demonstrated with MCF-7 and Br10 human breast cancer xenografts in nude mice. Osborne *et al.*[4] compared the antitumour effects of Faslodex and tamoxifen in a system that used estrogen-dependent human MCF-7 breast cancer cells growing in athymic nude mice. The authors observed that Faslodex was a more effective estrogen antagonist than tamoxifen. Furthermore, Hu *et al.*[5] showed that Faslodex completely circumvented tamoxifen resistance at a concentration of $5-10 \times 10^{-9}$ M using a tamoxifen-resistant MCF-7 cell line and suggested that the increased binding affinity for ER was a potential mechanism of action for their observations.

The antiuterotrophic potency of Faslodex was found to be 10-fold greater than that of tamoxifen in immature rats[1]. Using a rat model, Huynh *et al.*[6] reported that Faslodex decreased the uterine weight to 60% of controls and uterine IGF-I gene expression to 13% of controls compared with a 25% increase in uterine weight (125% of control) and 100% increase in IGF-I gene expression (200% of control) for tamoxifen. IGF-I is thought to, at least partly, mediate the uterotrophic effects of estradiol.

Clinical Studies

In a prospective randomized study of 56 postmenopausal women with operable breast cancer undergoing surgery, 37 patients were randomized to receive intramuscular Faslodex (6 mg or 18 mg) daily for 7 consecutive days prior to surgery. Defriend *et al.*[7] observed a significant decline in tumour ER expression in women who had received Faslodex. Furthermore the authors observed a significant decrease in Ki67 expression in ER-positive tumours but not in ER-negative tumours in women treated with preoperative Faslodex. Dixon *et al.* Have recently reported similar results[8]. The authors examined the effects of Faslodex on ER, PgR and Ki67 expression in postmenopausal women with previously untreated T1–T3 primary breast cancer. Faslodex (50 mg) significantly reduced the expression of ER, PgR and Ki67 compared with placebo. Furthermore, at a dose of 250 mg, Faslodex significantly decreased ER expression compared with tamoxifen (20 mg). Such results confirm that Faslodex downregulates ER expression and exhibits antiproliferative effects in postmenopausal women with ER-positive breast cancer. In another open randomized study in premenopausal women undergoing hysterectomy for benign endometrial disease, Thomas and colleagues[9] observed no effect of Faslodex on the hypothalamic–pituitary–gonadal axis.

Fulvestrant (Faslodex) was the focus of two main presentations during the 23rd San Antonio Breast Cancer Symposium (December 2000)[10,11]. Professor C. Kent Osborne[10] presented the results of the North American trial comparing Faslodex (250 mg once monthly) with anastrozole (Arimidex) in 400 postmenopausal women with advanced breast cancer (ABC) that had progressed or recurred on prior endocrine therapy. This was a double-blind, double-dummy, randomized multi-centre phase III trial. The authors observed no significant differences between Faslodex and Arimidex in terms of tolerability, median time to tumour progression (TTP) and objective response rate (18% and 17.5% respectively). However, the median duration of response was 9 months longer for the Faslodex group (19.3 versus 10.5 months). In a similar European trial[11] involving 451 postmenopausal women, the disease progressed in 83% of patients in each group. The median TTP, objective response rate, median duration of response, and tolerability were not significantly different between the two groups. The results of a combined analysis of both trials are awaited with interest. Such data suggest that Faslodex is at least as effective as Arimidex in postmenopausal women with hormone-sensitive ABC.

Administration and Adverse Effects

Faslodex is administered as a once-monthly intramuscular injection (250 mg in 5 ml). The local administration of this drug seems to be well-tolerated with less than 1% of patients reporting local tenderness and erythema. The adverse effects[10,11] include hot flushes (18%), gastrointestinal disturbances (40%), weight gain (0.5%) and vaginitis (0.5%).

EM-652 HCl

This is another pure antiestrogen with antiestrogenic activity in the mammary gland and the endometrium. Preclinical animal studies showed that this drug was a more potent inhibitor of tumour growth than tamoxifen, toremifene, droloxifene, idoxifene or raloxifene[11]. Furthermore, initial results also suggested favourable effects on bone density and lipids profile. Future clinical trials will clarify the potential role of this drug in the treatment and prevention of breast cancer.

References

1. Nawaz Z, Stancel GM, Hyder SM. The pure antiestrogen ICI 182,780 inhibits progestin-induced transcription. *Cancer Res* 1999; **59**: 372–376.
2. Huynh H, Nickerson T, Pollak M *et al.* Regulation of insulin-like growth factor I receptor expression by the pure antiestrogen ICI 182780. *Clin Cancer Res* 1996; **2**: 2037–2042.
3. Wakeling AE, Dukes M, Bowler J. A potent specific pure antiestrogen with clinical potential. *Cancer Res* 1991; **51**: 3867–3873.
4. Osbornc CK, Coronado-Heinsohn EB, Hilsenbeck SG *et al.* Comparison of the effects of a pure steroidal antiestrogen with those of tamoxifen in a model of human breast cancer. *J Natl Cancer* 1995; **87**: 746–750.
5. Hu XF, Veroni M, De Luise M *et al.* Circumvention of tamoxifen resistance by the pure antiestrogen ICI 182,780. *Int J Cancer* 1993; **55**: 873–876.
6. Huynh HT, Pollak M. Insulin-like growth factor I gene expression in the uterus is stimulated by tamoxifen and inhibited by the pure antiestrogen ICI 182780. *Cancer Res* 1993; **53**: 5585–5588.
7. Defriend DJ, Howell A, Nicholson RI *et al.* Investigation of a new pure antiestrogen (ICI 182,780) in women with primary breast cancer. *Cancer Res* 1994; **54**: 408–414.
8. Dixon JM, Nicholson RI, Robertson JFR *et al.* Comparison of the short-term biological effects of fulvestrant (ICI 182,780) with tamoxifen in postmenopausal women with primary breast cancer. *Eur J Cancer* 2000; **36**: S73.
9. Thomas EJ, Walton PL, Thomas NM *et al.* The effects of ICI 182,780, a pure antiestrogen, on the hypothalamic–pituitary–gonadal axis and on endometrial proliferation in premenopausal women. *Hum Reprod* 1994; **9**: 1991–1996.
10. Osborne CK, Pippen J, Parker L, *et al.* A double-blind randomized trial comparing the efficacy and tolerability of Faslodex (fulvestrant) with Arimidex (anastrozole) in postmenopausal women with advanced breast cancer. *Breast Cancer Res Treat* 2000; **64**: 27.

11. Howell A, Robertson JFR, Quaresma Albano J, *et al.* Comparison of efficacy and tolerability of fulvestrant (Faslodex) with anastrozole (Arimidex) in postmenopausal women with advanced breast cancer – preliminary results. *Breast Cancer Res Treat* 2000; **64**: 27.

12. Couillard S, Gutman M, Roy J *et al.* Comparison of the effects of EM-652.HCL (SCH.57068HCL), tamoxifen, toremifene, droloxifene, idoxifene, GW-5638 and raloxifene on the growth of human ZR-75-1 breast tumor in nude mice. *Proc Am Soc Clin Oncol* 2000; **76a**: Abstr. 292.

8. Ovarian Ablation

K. Kirkpatrick and K. Mokbel

Introduction

In July 1896, George Beatson published the first report of ovarian ablation for advanced breast cancer[1]. In 1959, Paterson and Russell reported
the first randomized trial evaluating ovarian ablation as an adjuvant
treatment for early breast cancer[2]. Subsequently several trials examined
the role of ovarian ablation in patients with the disease.

Ovarian Ablation by Surgery or Radiotherapy

The role of ovarian ablation by irradiation or surgery was examined by
at least 12 clinical trials that commenced before 1990. In 1995, the Early
Breast Cancer Trialists' Collaboration Group (EBCTCG) conducted a
meta-analysis of these 12 randomized trials[3]. The trials included 3456
patients (2102 women < 50 years and 1354 women ≥50 years) who
were accrued during 1984–1989. Ovarian ablation was achieved by
radiation in 7 of 12 studies. The dose ranged from 450 to 2000 rads.
Adjuvant cytotoxic chemotherapy was used in five studies that included
1144 women. Prednisolone was added to radiotherapy in two trials.
Data on ER status was only available in five trials. The follow-up period
exceeded 15 years for most patients. For women younger than 50 years
at the time of randomization, the disease free survival (DFS) at 15 years
was 45% for the ovarian ablation group versus 39% for the control arm
(Figure 1). For overall survival the absolute benefit of ovarian ablation
was 6.3% (52.4 vs 46.1%, $p = 0.0005$). Furthermore, the survival benefit was greater for patients with node-positive disease in the absence of
chemotherapy. Subgroup analysis also showed that ovarian ablation
produced greater improvement in DFS (25 vs 10%) and overall survival

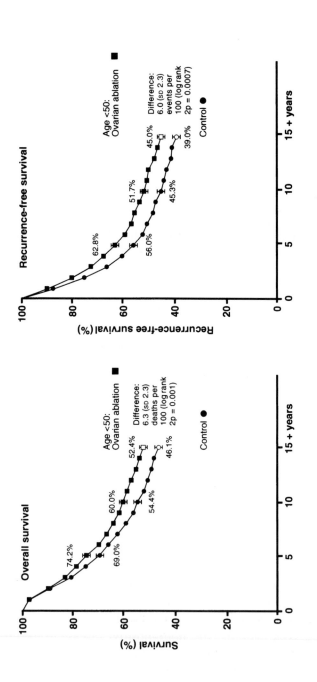

Figure 1 Kaplan–Meier survival curves for the effects of ovarian ablation on survival in women younger than 50 years (meta-analysis of 12 randomized trials, *n* = 2102)

(24 vs 8%) in the absence of chemotherapy. However, this difference failed to reach statistical significance, probably due to the small sample size. Therefore it is difficult to determine the benefit of chemotherapy due to induced ovarian suppression. The ER status was known in trials that used chemotherapy. Ovarian ablation showed no traditional benefit to chemotherapy in women with ER-poor tumours ($n = 194$). In women with ER-positive tumours, ovarian ablation improved DFS and overall survival by 13% and 17% respectively.

It can be concluded from the EBCTCG overview that ovarian ablation significantly improves DFS and overall survival in premenopausal women. However, the data were insufficient to reliably assess the importance of ER and whether ovarian ablation offers significant additional benefit compare with cytotoxic therapy.

Surgical oophorectomy is nowadays performed using laparoscopic techniques. Laparoscopic oophorectomy has been shown to be safe and well tolerated and is currently considered as part of the management of ER-positive premenopausal breast cancer[4].

Goserelin (Zoladex)

Goserelin (Zoladex) is a decapeptide agonist at the luteinizing hormone releasing hormone (LHRH) receptor. It is the most widely studied LHRH analogue. The drug suppresses ovarian function in premenopausal and peri-menopausal women to castration levels after initial stimulation. Goserelin is given by subcutaneous injection (3.6 mg) every 28 days. It is well tolerated and the main side-effects are related to ovarian suppression and are reversible after cessation of treatment.

Goserelin in Advanced Breast Cancer

Several studies have demonstrated objective response in 36% of patients with stage III or IV breast cancer after treatment with goserelin 3.6 mg subcutaneously every 28 days. Furthermore, another 50% of patients showed stabilization of the disease[5,6]. The median duration of response was 44 weeks. Taylor *et al.* compared Zoladex directly with surgical oophorectomy in 136 premenopausal women with metastatic breast cancer with no previous chemotherapy or hormonal treatment[7]. All tumours were either ER or PgR-positive. Objective response was observed in 27% of patients undergoing surgical ovarian ablation compared with 31% of patients receiving Zoladex.

The median overall survival of the Zoladex group was 37 months compared with 33 months for the surgical ovarian ablation group. Furthermore, the authors observed that Zoladex reduced serum estradiol levels to postmenopausal levels.

Zoladex and Early Breast Cancer

The role of Zoladex in the adjuvant setting for early breast cancer in premenopausal women is currently being investigated by several clinical trials. The Cancer Research Campaign (CRC) is conducting a four-arm trial, known as the ZIPP trial (2×2 factorial design). Patients are randomized into Zoladex alone, tamoxifen alone, Zoladex plus tamoxifen or no further treatment[8]. Administration of chemotherapy is not an exclusion criterion. Seventy-one percent of patients recruited so far are ER-positive and the ER status has not been determined in 25% of cases. The initial analysis at 5 years of 2648 patients participating in the study showed that Zoladex was associated with prolonged disease-free survival (RR = 0.75, $p = 0.001$). However, the improvement in overall survival failed to reach statistical significance (RR = 0.78, $p = 0.08$). Furthermore, Zoladex decreased the risk of developing contralateral breast cancer by 40% ($p = 0.005$).

Other ongoing trials examining the adjuvant role of Zoladex in breast cancer include the International Breast Cancer Study Group VIII trial I (in which patients are randomized to receive Zoladex alone, six cycles of CMF or Zoladex plus CMF), The Eastern Co-operative Oncology Group and South Western Oncology Group (in which patients are randomized to six cycles of CAF, six cycles of CAF plus Zoladex for 5 years or six cycles of CAF plus 5 years of Zoladex and tamoxifen) and the Zoladex Early Breast Cancer Research Association (ZEBRA) trial (six cycles of CMF versus 2 years of Zoladex). Professor W. Jonal has recently presented the first efficacy results from the ZEBRA study in which 1640 node-positive patients aged less than 50 years were randomized to 3.6 mg of Zoladex for 2 years ($n = 817$) or six cycles of CMF ($n = 823$). In ER-positive patients (73% of the study population), Zoladex was equivalent to CMF in terms of DFS (HR = 1, 95% CI = 0.83–1.20) without the distressing side-effects associated with cytotoxic chemotherapy[9].

Laparoscopic Oophorectomy

Technique

The patient is placed supine on the operating table under general anaesthesia with endotracheal intubation and ventilation. Placing the patient in the Lloyd–Davies position is useful in allowing intra-operative anteversion of the uterus using a speculum to bring the ovaries into view. Full preparation of the abdominal skin is performed and surgical drapes applied to expose the surgical field.

A pneumoperitoneum is created to a pressure of 15–20 mmHg using carbon dioxide through a Verres needle. This is inserted at right angles to the skin, most commonly through a vertical or transverse skin incision at the lower edge of the umbilicus, this being where the abdominal wall is at its thinnest. Prior to piercing the rectus sheath the abdominal wall is elevated, either manually or by placing sutures into the fascia, to increase the distance of the needle from intra-abdominal structures. The presence of previous abdominal scars in the area may require insertion of the Verres needle at a point distant to the area in order to allow the safe creation of a pneumoperitoneum and visualization of the peritoneal cavity with the camera prior to continuing with surgery. Alternatively the abdominal wall may be opened under direct vision through an incision large enough to accommodate a trocar for insufflation. Confirmation of peritoneal entry can be established by observing that saline in a syringe drains freely through the needle hub and cannot then be aspirated, or by using a needle designed to produce an audible click on passing through the abdominal wall and the peritoneum.

Once a tense pneumoperitoneum is established, an incision is made through the abdominal wall fascia to allow insertion of a 10 mm trocar, which should be introduced with a steady pressure aiming towards the anus and kept in the midline to avoid the sacral promontory and overlying aorta and the pelvic vessels. On entry into the peritoneal cavity, the trocar can be removed and the gas outlet tube connected to the port. The abdominal viscera can now be visualized with the laparoscope and further ports inserted as shown (Figure 2). When the ports have been inserted, applying head-down tilt to the operating table ensures movement of the bowel out of the pelvis.

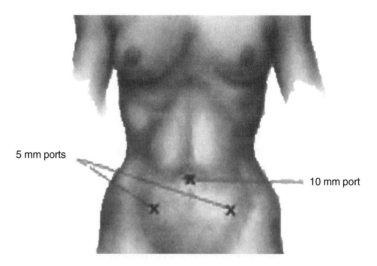

Figure 2   Port sites for laparoscopic oophorectomy

The internal genitalia are inspected and the ureter identified. A pair of grasping forceps is inserted through one of the smaller ports and is used to pull the ovary medially and display the mesovarium. The infundibulo-pelvic ligament is either clipped in its entirety before division or skeletonized by dissection through the broad ligament to expose the ovarian vessels, which are then clipped. Following removal of both ovaries in this manner the ports are removed and the pneumoperitoneum released. The abdominal wall fascia at the site of the large port insertion is closed with a slowly absorbable or non-absorbable suture to prevent incisional hernias and the skin closed as desired.

Complications

Specific complications of this operation are the risks of inadequate ligation of the ovarian pedicle, with subsequent haemorrhage, and damage to the ureter, bowel or bladder. Other complications apply to laparoscopic surgery in general, and include the risks in creating a pneumoperitoneum and the risks involved in the blind insertion of the initial trocar.

A tense pneumoperitoneum causes a reduction in venous return and an increase in central venous and intrathoracic pressures, which can compromise patients with cardiovascular disease. The increased intra-abdominal pressure leads to a risk of regurgitation of gastric contents. Gas embolism can occur if the Verres needle is inserted into a blood vessel, or if gas enters through a torn vessel – particularly in the Trendelenburg position, where there is a pressure gradient from the pelvic vessels to the heart. Deaths from gas embolism are rare using carbon dioxide because of its solubility, although absorption will cause hypercarbia.

Damage to the aorta or pelvic vessels can occur, most commonly during the initial trocar insertion. The inferior epigastric vessels can be damaged during insertion of the secondary ports, and care should be taken to visualize these vessels directly with the laparoscope or by transillumination.

The bowel is vulnerable to damage from diathermy and from trocar insertion, particularly if adhesions are present. The bladder is susceptible to damage by Verres needles and trocars, more so if preoperative catheterization has not been performed.

References

1. Beatson GT. On the treatment of inoperable cases of carcinoma of the mamma: suggestions for a new treatment with illustrative cases. *Lancet* 1896; **iii**: 104–107.
2. Paterson R, Russell MH. Clinical trials in malignant disease, part II. Breast cancer, value of irradiation of the ovaries. *J Fac Radiol* 1959; **10**: 130–133.
3. Early Breast Cancer Trialists' Collaborative Group. Ovarian ablation in early breast cancer; overview of the randomised trials. *Lancet* 1996; **348**: 1189–1196.
4. O'Boyle CJ, O'Hanlon DM, Kerin MJ *et al.* Laparoscopic oophorectomy, a prospective evaluation in premenopausal breast cancer with particular reference to incidence and severity of menopausal symptoms. *Eur J Surg Oncol* 1996; **22**: 491–493.
5. Milstad RAV, Matthew MJ. A review of the international experience with the LHRH agonist 'Zoladex' in the treatment of advanced breast cancer in pre and perimenopausal women. In Gholdhirsch A ed. *European School of Oncology (ESO) Monography Series* 1990; *Endocrine Therapy of Breast Cancer IV*: 59–65.
6. Blamey RW, Jonat W, Kaumann M *et al.* Goserelin depot in the treatment of premenopausal advanced breast cancer. *Eur J Cancer* 1992; **28A**: 810–814.
7. Taylor CW, Green S, Dalton WS *et al.* Multicenter randomised clinical trial of goserelin versus surgical ovariectomy in premenopausal patients with receptor-positive metastatic breast cancer. *J Clin Oncol* 1998; **16**: 993–999.

8. Houghton J, Baum L, Rutqvist B *et al.* The ZIPP trial of adjuvant Zoladex in premenopausal patients with early breast cancer: An update at 5 years. *Proc Am Soc Clin Oncol* 2000; **93a**: Abstr 359.
9. Jonal W. Zoladex™ (goserelin) vs. CMF as adjuvant therapy in pre-/perimenopausal node-positive breast cancer: first efficacy results from the ZEBRA study. *Eur J Cancer* 2000; **36**: S67.

9. Chemoprevention

A. C. Leris and K. Mokbel

Introduction

Breast Cancer affects 1 in 12 British women and remains a leading cause of death. The belief that breast cancer may be a preventable disease is based upon strong epidemiological evidence. Incidence is associated with modifiable environmental and physiological variables, i.e. diet and serum estradiol respectively. Current avenues of research include the Selective Estrogen Receptor Modulators (SERMs), retinoids, dietary manipulation and vitamin supplementation. Animal studies show that mammary tumour incidence increases with fat intake, and suggest that fat acts as a promoter of carcinogenesis[1]. Dietary fat reduction and exercise have been shown to significantly reduce serum estradiol (-13.4%, meta-analysis of 13 dietary fat intervention studies[2]). However, there is no conclusive evidence that reduction in serum estradiol levels reduces the risk of breast cancer. The protective effect of exercise has been demonstrated in epidemiological studies[3].

Phytoestrogens may play a role in the reduced incidence of breast cancer seen in East Asia. Pre-pubertal exposure to phytoestrogens in rats reduces the incidence and multiplicity of induced mammary carcinomas[4]. Furthermore, incubation of human breast cancer cells with genistein (a phytoestrogen) causes cell growth inhibition and increasing differentiation[5] and treated cells behave less aggressively when xenografted to nude mice. However, a recent population study from Japan has failed to confirm benefit[6]. There is no evidence that vitamin supplementation reduces the risk of breast cancer. Wu *et al.* have recently reported that low levels of vitamin B_{12} in postmenopausal women are associated with an increased risk of breast cancer[7]. However, this study was a nested case–control study in which women with

69

postmenopausal breast cancer were found to have lower serum levels of vitamin B_{12} (although still within the normal range) than controls who were matched only by age, race and menopausal status.

There is increasing evidence that breast cancer risk correlates with raised levels of insulin-like growth factor-I (IGF-I)[8]. In a randomized study of 3000 women with early breast cancer, Fenretinide, a vitamin A derivative which reduces IGF-I levels, was found to significantly reduce the risk of contralateral breast cancer in premenopausal women; the risk, however, was increased in postmenopausal women[9]. Although there may be a biological rationale for this differential effect, it would be inappropriate to accept this finding at face value and further investigations are required to ensure that this observation is not a chance finding.

SERMs

The concept of an ideal antiestrogen was first proposed in 1990 at the Eighth Cain Memorial Award lecture[10]. This proposal has led to a new direction in drug development which has culminated in the drugs known today as selective estrogen receptor modulators (SERMs). The ideal SERM would have beneficial estrogen-like and antiestrogenic properties. In brief it would have the positive characteristics associated with HRT, reducing ischaemic heart disease, preventing menopausal vasomotor and emotional symptoms whilst maintaining bone density and libido. It would have antiestrogenic effects in the breast and uterus, reducing the incidence of malignancy, without thrombotic complications. This ideal drug has yet to be found.

Tamoxifen

Tamoxifen, a non-steroidal antiestrogen is the most thoroughly evaluated of the selective estrogen receptor modulators. In the breast, it completely inhibits the binding of estrogen to estrogen receptors. This affects the expression of estrogen-regulated genes that influence G1 growth arrest and apoptosis. It has been licensed for the treatment of breast cancer since 1978 and for the chemoprevention of breast cancer in the USA since 1998.

NSABP-P1 Study

In 1992, the National Surgical Adjuvant Breast and Bowel Project (NSABP) launched a randomized clinical trial of tamoxifen for the prevention of breast cancer[11]. Secondary aims were to determine whether tamoxifen would lower the incidence of myocardial infarction and bony fractures. It would also assess the impact of tamoxifen on healthy women with particular reference to the incidence of endometrial cancer and pulmonary embolism. Tamoxifen was chosen because it had a proven track record in the treatment of breast cancer, there was already evidence to suggest that prevention with this agent was a real possibility. The main evidence came from trials of adjuvant tamoxifen therapy for stage I and II breast cancer. A recent overview[12] of 55 trials of adjuvant tamoxifen therapy involving 37 000 women and 87% of the world-wide evidence on tamoxifen showed that in trials of 1, 2 and 5 years of therapy, the proportional reductions in the incidence of contralateral breast cancer were 13% (SD 13; NS), 26% (SD 9; $2p = 0.004$) and 47% (SD 9; $2p < 0.0001$) respectively (Figure 1). The tendency of trials of longer tamoxifen duration to involve larger reductions in the incidence of new primary cancer in the opposite breast is significant (trend test $\chi^2 = 7.3$; $2p < 0.008$). These results indicate that tamoxifen halves the annual incidence of contralateral breast cancer. The proportional risk reductions were independent of age, and appeared to be the same for women with ER-poor tumours. The NSABP

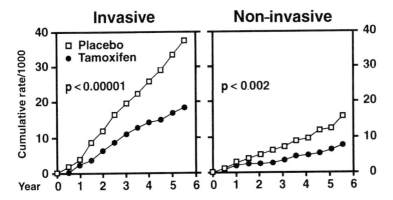

Figure 1 Cumulative rates of invasive and non-invasive breast cancer in the tamoxifen and placebo groups in the NSABP-P1 trial ($n = 13\ 175$)

P-1 trial was launched in the US through 131 centres, randomization began in June 1992. Each centre had on-site auditing to monitor and assess data quality.

Eligibility for the study was defined as a risk >1.66% per year of developing breast cancer (the risk for a 60-year-old woman with no additional risk factors). This was assessed using a modified Gail model which used multivariate logistic regression analysis to assign risk based on accepted risk factors for breast cancer. These include age, number of first-degree relatives with breast cancer, nulliparity or age at first birth, number of breast biopsies, diagnosis of atypical hyperplasia and age at menarche. The original Gail model incorporated the expected incidence of ductal carcinoma in situ (DCIS), it was modified for the purposes of this study to give the expected rates of invasive breast cancer only, using data from the SEER study. Women with a previous history of lobular carcinoma in situ (LCIS) were also eligible. The participants had to have a life expectancy of greater than 10 years and no mammographic or clinical evidence of breast cancer at randomization. After July 1994, all patients underwent endometrial sampling in addition to other tests on entry. No participants were able to take hormonal therapy during the trial and intent to become pregnant or history of DVT/PE were absolute exclusion criteria. Randomization was double blind and participants were stratified by age, race, history of LCIS and relative risk of breast cancer as computed by the modified Gail model. The trial was independently monitored. 13 388 women were randomized to receive either tamoxifen 20 mg daily or placebo. 13 175 women were included in the final analysis of follow-up data from accrual to March 31, 1998 which was the day before the trial was unblinded. Mean follow-up was 47.7 months.

Results

A total of 368 invasive and non-invasive breast cancers occurred amongst the 13 175 participants, 244 in the placebo group and 124 in the tamoxifen group. There was a highly significant reduction in the incidence of breast cancer in the tamoxifen group. The disease was observed both for the incidence of invasive and non-invasive disease. For invasive breast cancer there was a 49% reduction in the overall risk ($p < 0.0001$). For non-invasive breast cancer the reduction in risk was 50% ($p < 0.002$). No survival difference between the two groups was

Table 1 Sub-group analysis in the NSABP P-1 trial of breast cancer prevention with tamoxifen

Subgroup characteristic	Rate per 1000 women		Risk ratio
	Placebo	*Tamoxifen*	
Age (yrs)			
<49	6.70	3.77	0.56
50–59	6.28	3.10	0.49
>60	7.33	3.33	0.45
History of LCIS			
No	6.41	3.30	0.51
Yes	12.99	5.69	0.44
Atypical hyperplasia			
No	6.44	3.61	0.56
Yes	10.11	1.43	0.14
5-year predicted risk			
<2.00	5.54	2.06	0.37
2.01–3.00	5.18	3.51	0.68
3.01–5.00	5.88	3.88	0.66
>5.01	13.28	4.52	0.34
Affected 1st-degree relatives			
0	6.45	2.97	0.46
1	6.00	3.03	0.51
2	8.68	4.75	0.55
>3	13.72	7.02	0.51
TOTAL	**6.76**	**3.43**	**0.51**

observed. Nine deaths were attributed to breast cancer, six in the placebo group and three in the tamoxifen group. Subgroup analysis showed that risk reduction occurred across all groups. This was particularly noticeable in the group with atypical hyperplasia, however, numbers in this subgroup were small (Table 1).

Risk reduction increased with duration of therapy ($p < 0.00001$ for invasive breast cancer, and $p = 0.002$ for non-invasive breast cancer).

Tamoxifen reduced the incidence of ER-positive tumours only. There was no significant difference in the incidence of ER-negative tumours between the tamoxifen and placebo groups. The risk reduction

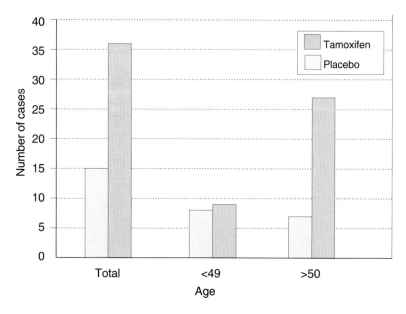

Figure 2   Increased risk of endometrial cancer in women taking tamoxifen

increased year on year through the study. After 1 year of treatment the reduction was 33% increasing to 69% at year 5. Reduced incidence of all sizes of tumour and both node-positive and negative tumours was seen.

The association between tamoxifen and endometrial cancer was confirmed. The relative risk for endometrial cancer in women taking tamoxifen was 2.53. All endometrial cancers found in the study group were grade one and there was no excess mortality from this cause (Figure 2). Patients taking tamoxifen are advised to contact their doctors if they develop abnormal vaginal bleeding, otherwise routine screening tests for endometrial cancer such as endometrial biopsies and ultrasonography are not worthwhile.

Side-effects

Less than 10% of women discontinued treatment and no differences in weight gain or depression was found between the groups. The risk of hot flushes was increased in treated women, however there was not a significant drop-out rate for this reason. It can be assumed that the

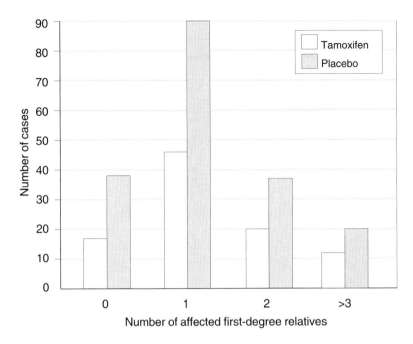

Figure 3 Effect of tamoxifen on women with a family history of breast cancer

side-effects of therapy are justified in the minds of motivated women at high risk of breast cancer.

Family History

BRCA 1/2 patients were involved in the study although laboratory analysis of gene status was not available at the time of analysis. It can be seen from the sub-group analysis provided that women involved in the trial as a consequence of strong family history did benefit from tamoxifen (Figure 3).

The Marsden Study

The Marsden study began in 1986[13]. It was a randomized double-blind placebo-controlled trial of tamoxifen for the prevention of breast cancer. A total of 2494 women have been recruited. Criteria for inclusion include one first-degree relative aged under 50, one first-degree relative

Table 2   Events during follow-up

	Tamoxifen	Placebo
Breast cancer	34	36
Other cancers	19	24
endometrial	4	1
ovarian	2	5
gastrointestinal	3	3
other	10	15
Deep vein thrombosis	4	2
Pulmonary embolism	3	2
Deaths		
Breast cancer	4	1
Other causes	5	5

of any age with bilateral breast cancer or one first-degree relative plus another first or second-degree relative of any age with breast cancer.

Women who were considering pregnancy, taking oral contraceptives, or had a history of deep vein thrombosis or pulmonary embolism were excluded.

So far 2471 women have been randomized to either tamoxifen 20 mg once daily or placebo. All participants had no evidence of breast cancer on randomization and were regularly screened.

Results

Women were analysed by intention to treat. Both groups were well matched for age and menopausal status. Median follow-up stands at 70 months and 70 breast cancers have occurred in the cohort.

This study has so far shown no preventative effect for tamoxifen (Table 2).

A total of 877 women have stopped the trial because of side-effects (tamoxifen 320, placebo 176; $p = 0.0005$). The most frequently reported side-effects were hot flushes/vasomotor problems, menstrual irregularities, vaginal discharge and benign abnormalities found on transvaginal ultrasound. 649 women took HRT during the trial; they were evenly split between the treatment and placebo groups.

This trial has high power (90%) to detect an effect for tamoxifen in the prevention of breast cancer. There was good compliance (78%

confirmed by subset blood sampling). There is also good evidence that tamoxifen had other effects in these women including lowering serum cholesterol. However the study population differed greatly from those women in the NSABP trial and from most women with breast cancer. Entry criteria were based on a family history of breast cancer. It is likely that this study group had a far higher prevalence of BRCA 1/2 and other mutations yet to be described than any other population for whom we have data on tamoxifen therapy. The investigators estimate from pedigree analysis that approximately 60% of the women who developed breast cancer during the trial have a breast cancer susceptibility gene and that 36% of the study population as a whole have a breast cancer susceptibility gene. It has been suggested that the estrogen promotion required for most sporadic cancers of the breast is not required in genetic type cancer, or that at this early stage, when estrogen receptors are present and where antiestrogens may exert their influence, it is truncated or absent in genetic cancers. Evidence for this theory includes the increased frequency of ER-negative tumours in these women. Indeed the breast cancer susceptibility gene may code for some abnormality of estrogen receptors, which cause abnormal function and enhance the chance of developing malignancy.

Although it appears from retrospective histopathological studies that breast cancers arising in BRCA 1 mutation carriers are most likely to be ER-negative, there is evidence that bilateral oophorectomy significantly reduces the breast cancer risk in BRCA 1 carriers[14], thus complicating the above theory.

Follow-up of these women continues. The same team has instituted a second placebo-controlled trial of toremifene and trials of idoxifene are likely to start soon.

The International Breast Cancer Intervention Study (IBIS) trial also continues; this mainly European study requires a sample of 7000 women, who will be randomized to 5 years of tamoxifen or placebo. A recent questionnaire survey of participants in Manchester showed that women were aware that longer follow-up to fully assess the risk–benefit ratio was required and no one has dropped out of this trial as a result of the early publication of the American NSABP trial results[15].

The Italian Study

The Italian study interim analysis[16] again showed no effect for tamoxifen in the reduction of breast cancer incidence except in those women who had taken HRT. The interim data were presented in July 1998 in response to the publication of the NSABP P-1 trial discussed above.

The study was a double-blind, multicentre, randomized placebo-controlled trial. There were 55 centres involved in recruitment and follow-up, the vast majority being in Italy. 5408 women were randomized, and data have been analysed on intention to treat. These women were mainly at relatively low to normal risk of breast cancer. However 18.2% had at least one first-degree relative with breast cancer.

All participants had had a hysterectomy for benign disease, and most had also had bilateral oophorectomy.

Overall 1027 women have dropped out of the study (301 because of side-effects), and 239 have withdrawn because of adverse events. 149 have completed 5 years of treatment and 3837 are still being treated. The median duration of follow-up is 46 months and continues. However, recruitment has been terminated early because of problems with poor compliance.

Results

There were no significant differences between the incidence, type, size or receptor status of the breast cancers developing in the tamoxifen-treated or placebo groups. No deaths from breast cancer have been observed in the study population. Of women taking HRT throughout the trial (752), nine developed breast cancer, eight in the placebo group and one in the tamoxifen group ($p = 0.0216$).

Adverse events associated with tamoxifen therapy included 64 thrombotic or embolic events, 42 being superficial phlebitis. Of these, 18 occurred in the placebo group and 38 in the tamoxifen group ($p = 0.0053$). There were 14 documented strokes, five in the placebo arm and nine in the tamoxifen arm of the trial ($p = 0.27$). Hypertriglyceridaemia was not formally measured in the study, but it was reported as occurring in 17 women in the study – 15 on tamoxifen and two on placebo ($p = 0.0013$).

The investigators stopped recruiting to the study mainly because large numbers of women withdrew because of secondary side-effects from tamoxifen. The number of vascular events, in combination with the unexpected findings of hypertriglyceridaemia, provided further incentive. Follow-up of these women continues. The power of this study to detect an effect of tamoxifen in preventing breast cancer is small but will increase as follow-up of the women being treated grows. The data on tamoxifen and HRT requires further investigation.

Weighing Individual Risks in the Decision to Take Tamoxifen

In July 1998, the National Cancer Institute sponsored a workshop[17], the principal aim of which was to develop guidelines based on risk analysis to help women decide whether or not to take tamoxifen to prevent breast cancer. Information from all trials on the risks and benefits of tamoxifen were reviewed. Other health outcomes for women in the relevant age groups in the absence of tamoxifen were also reviewed. They concluded that the risks and benefits of tamoxifen therapy depended on each individual woman's risk factors for breast cancer and other health problems, including ischaemic heart disease and thromboembolic problems. They pointed out that the absolute risk of endometrial cancer, stroke, pulmonary embolism, and deep vein thrombosis increases with age and this effect is compounded by tamoxifen therapy. However this effect is tempered by the relative risk reduction from fractures and breast cancer. They have produced risk analysis tables which can be tailored to each woman depending upon the value she would place on each individual side-effect of tamoxifen and suggest that these tables could be used as tools to enable physicians and patients to make informed decisions about tamoxifen chemoprevention.

It is well known that women with a history of DCIS, LCIS, BRCA 1 and 2, Cowden's and Li–Fraumeni syndromes are at higher risk of breast cancer. These factors are not taken into consideration using the Gail model and therefore increased weight should be given to these predisposing factors in addition to those factors used for computing risk in the Gail model (which forms the basis for risk stratification in the tables). Similarly protective factors, such as oriental origin, should also be taken into consideration. Increased tendency towards ischaemic

Table 3 **Individual factors relevant to increased risk of side-effects from tamoxifen therapy**

Outcome	Factors	Effect on risk (relative risk)
Endometrial cancer	Unopposed estrogen replacement >10 yrs	↑ (5–10)
	Nulliparity; obesity; menopause >55yrs	↑(2)
	Diabetes, ↑BP	↑(?2° to obesity)
	Estrogen with progestins	Little risk
	Oral contraceptives	↓(0.5)
	Current smoking	↓(0.5)
Stroke	Transient ischaemic attacks	↑(5–30) esp. older women
	Mitral valve disease, AF	↑(2.5)
	Smoking, IHD, ↑BP, DM	↑
	Oral contraceptives, pregnancy, SLE	↑
Pulmonary embolism or deep vein thrombosis	Trauma/surgery, immobility, pregnancy, smoking, obesity, oral contraceptives	↑

heart disease and stroke would act as relative contraindications to tamoxifen therapy. For women with a uterus, the relative risk of endometrial cancer is a further complicating factor. Tables of risk modification by individual characteristics have been constructed (see Table 3).

Tables of net/benefit risk for women stratified by age and risk of developing breast cancer have been constructed (Table 4).

Table 4 shows the relative risk of adverse events whilst taking tamoxifen. Examination of the column for women aged 40–49 shows that women are positively and negatively affected by taking tamoxifen (for 5 years per 10 000 women). It can be seen that 97 women would avoid breast cancer but 16 would develop endometrial cancer. All events in the 'Life threatening' category have been weighted[1]. This gives an overall survival advantage of 54/10 000 women taking tamoxifen. The 'Severe' events have been weighted 0.5 and these therefore give an overall survival advantage for 19/10 000 women taking tamoxifen. Other

Table 4 Net benefit/risk of tamoxifen therapy – see text for explanation

Severity of event	Type of event	White women 2.0% risk of invasive breast cancer Age 40–49 yrs	Age 50–59 yrs
Life threatening	Invasive breast cancer	97	97
	Hip fracture	1	22
	Endometrial cancer	−16	−120
	Stroke	−13	−32
	Pulmonary embolism	−15	−49
Severe	*In situ* breast cancer	53	31
	Deep vein thrombosis	−15	−16
Other	Colles fracture	11	19
	Spine fracture	2	23
	Cataracts	−35	−101
Net benefit/risk index, with uterus (1, 0.5, 0)		**73**	**−75**
Net benefit/risk index, without uterus (1, 0.5, 0)		**89**	**46**

events have been included in the table but are weighted 0. This gives an overall survival advantage for 73/10 000 women from taking tamoxifen for 5 years in the 40–49 age group with a 2% 5-year risk of developing breast cancer. However, if the same data are computed for women of the same age with a 4% 5-year risk of developing breast cancer, then the survival advantage increases to 196 with the same weighting. The greatest survival advantage from taking tamoxifen is seen in women aged 40–49 with a 6% risk of developing breast cancer over 5 years and no uterus – 334/10 000 women avoid life threatening events. Gain is reduced to 318/10 000 women for those with a uterus due to the projected 120 cases of endometrial cancer. However it is as well to bear in mind that all excess cases of endometrial cancer in the NSABP P-1 trial were stage 1, with no deaths from this cause.

Special consideration was given to BRCA 1/2 mutation carriers. It has been demonstrated that these women have a 37–85% life-time risk of developing invasive breast cancer, and therefore they would be ideal candidates for breast cancer chemoprevention. However no data exist on the effectiveness of this strategy. They also have a preponderance to develop ER-poor tumours. Furthermore the Royal Marsden study showed no effect for tamoxifen chemoprevention and this study probably contained the highest number of women carrying these mutations, bearing in mind the inclusion criteria. The current advice in the States is to offer these women prevention in the form of tamoxifen with the proviso that it may prove to be ineffective.

Monitoring of Women on Tamoxifen

Most evidence on the appropriate monitoring of women on tamoxifen comes from the NSABP P-1 study. No haematological or hepatic toxicity has been reported with tamoxifen and therefore screening blood tests are not required. It is still unclear whether routine screening for endometrial cancer should be carried out, however current recommendations from the American College of Obstetricians and Gynecologists include annual pelvic ultrasound examination and PAP smears. All women should be counselled about the endometrial effects of tamoxifen and any abnormal vaginal bleeding investigated, usually by endometrial biopsy.

Women should be counselled about visual side-effects and symptoms of visual disturbance elicited during follow-up visits should be appropriately investigated.

Raloxifene

Raloxifene is the second most well-evaluated SERM. Its use as a preventative agent for breast cancer is currently being evaluated. Evidence for its preventive effect comes from the Multiple Outcomes of Raloxifene Trial (MORE) study[18]. This was mainly designed to quantify the risk reduction for fractures in women with osteoporosis (licensed indication for raloxifene). Women with osteoporosis are at reduced risk of breast cancer anyway. Further work is required in women at higher risk of breast cancer who would be suitable in terms of risk/benefit analysis to take a SERM for this indication.

The MORE study was a 3-year randomized placebo-controlled trial involving 7705 women with osteoporosis. This was defined by the pres-

Table 5 Results of the MORE trial

	Placebo	Raloxifene (combined groups)	Relative risk (95% CI)
No. of subjects	2576	5129	
Invasive breast cancer	27	13	0.24 (0.13–0.44)
All breast cancer	32	22	0.35 (0.21–0.58)
ER-positive breast cancer	20	4	0.10 (0.04–0.24)
ER-negative breast cancer	4	7	0.88 (0.26–3.00)
Endometrial cancer	4	6	$p = 0.67$
Deep vein thrombosis	5	18	RR=3.1 (1.5–6.2) $p = 0.002$
Pulmonary embolism	3	10	RR=3.1 (1.5–6.2) $p = 0.08$
Hot flushes	165	548	$p = <0.001$

ence of vertebral fractures, and a femoral neck or spine T-score of at least 2.5 SDs below the mean for young healthy women. Women taking estrogens or with a history of breast cancer were excluded.

Women were randomized to take raloxifene 60 mg once or twice daily, or one or two placebo tablets. All women were screened using mammography or breast ultrasound at 0, 2 and 3 years (year 1 was optional).

Raloxifene reduced the risk of newly diagnosed breast cancer during the study by 76% over a median of 40 months' treatment. As with tamoxifen, the main reduction was seen in the incidence of ER-positive tumours in the treatment group (RR = 0.1, i.e. 90% reduction in ER-positive tumours). There was no significant increase in the incidence of endometrial cancer (Table 5). In fact the results of this trial suggest that no monitoring of the endometrium is required for women on raloxifene. Increased rates of thromboembolic disease correlate with those of tamoxifen in the NASBP trial of chemoprevention.

If the risk reduction in terms of prevention of breast cancer was of the same magnitude or greater than that seen with tamoxifen in higher risk women as in the NSABP trial, this suggests that raloxifene would be the most ideal SERM for breast cancer prevention so far. However women in the MORE and NSABP trial of prevention of breast cancer are not directly comparable because women with osteoporosis are at reduced risk of breast cancer. Tamoxifen has not been tested in low-risk women; it has been hypothesized that its effect would be even greater in this sub-group. The women in the MORE trial were also older than the participants in the NSABP and Marsden trials. However the results do suggest that raloxifene may be useful for the combined reduction of ER-positive breast cancer and vertebral fractures in older women. Although raloxifene does increase menopausal symptoms they are much less troublesome than those seen with tamoxifen. This fact, in conjunction with its antiestrogenic effects on the uterus, may make raloxifene the ideal SERM, particularly in the older lower-risk patient.

Since breast cancer risk reduction was a secondary endpoint in the MORE study, the multiplicity issue therefore remains a source of bias in this study and the results of the NSABP-P2 trials are likely to clarify the potential role of raloxifene in chemoprevention.

The Study of Tamoxifen and Raloxifene (STAR) trial aims to directly compare the effect of raloxifene and tamoxifen in the prevention of breast cancer. It will be conducted on 22 000 postmenopausal women. Eligibility criteria are otherwise similar to the NSABP trial of breast cancer prevention. Subjects are randomly assigned to 5 years' treatment with either tamoxifen 20 mg daily, or raloxifene 60 mg daily. It is thought that raloxifene will have a higher therapeutic index than tamoxifen mainly because of the reduced incidence of endometrial cancer. Apart from this reduced incidence of endometrial cancer, the adverse event profile (mainly increased risk of thromboembolic disease) between the two drugs are similar. It is also likely that the therapeutic index for raloxifene will be higher in younger women at higher risk of breast cancer. To assess this effect hopefully premenopausal women will become eligible for this trial when evaluation data for raloxifene in this age group become available (evaluation on-going).

Prevention of Breast Cancer with SERMs

It is thought that, as a reduction in breast cancer incidence was seen so early in these trials, this was the result of treating sub-clinical breast cancer. It is unknown whether waiting until these cancers presented and treating them as they arose would result in a better or worse prognosis for affected women. It is known that metastatic breast cancers develop resistance to tamoxifen in the long term. It has also been shown that use of tamoxifen for longer than 5 years has no proven benefit to women in terms of prevention of new disease or progression of existing disease. It is unclear whether the chemoprevention of breast cancer with SERMs simply delays presentation of disease by an as yet unknown period of time or whether treating these cancers as they arose would have the same outcome. If tamoxifen simply reduces lead-time bias, when these women do present they will have an apparently worse outlook. Only very long-term follow-up can answer these questions. The NSABP trial showed a highly significant effect on the incidence of invasive and non-invasive breast cancer. The Italian study failed to show any effect, but compliance was extremely low and this is one of the main problems with this trial. In women who were compliant with therapy, there is a trend towards a preventive effect for tamoxifen. However this has not achieved significance as yet.

The Marsden study had vastly different recruitment criteria; it has been estimated from pedigree analysis that 37% of the women in the trial have some breast cancer predisposing gene. It is estimated that approximately 60% of women who developed breast cancer during the trial have a breast cancer predisposition gene. It is well accepted that BRCA 1/2 carriers develop ER-negative tumours. Initiation and promotion of malignant cells may follow a more accelerated progression in these women and may not involve an ER-positive phase as is thought to happen in most breast cancers. It is perhaps unsurprising that the Marsden study has failed to show a chemopreventive affect.

Retinoids – Fenretinide

Retinoids are one of the most studied non-SERM agents. They are natural and synthetic analogues of vitamin A. They have demonstrable antitumour effects in pre-clinical models. Fenretinide, a synthetic derivative of all trans-retinoic acid has relatively high activity and low toxicity compared to other retinoids in its class. Clinical studies have shown that it is accumulated in the human breast. This retinoid induces apoptosis, although its complete mechanism of action is unclear.

Veronesi *et al.*[9] performed a controlled trial of fenretinide in 2972 women aged 30–70 with early breast cancer. Patients were treated for 5 years with either fenretinide 200 mg daily or had no treatment. Unfortunately, as there was no placebo group in the trial, there are no accurate data on the side-effects or toxicity of fenretinide. However, compliance is reported as good and only 4.4% of the treated group discontinued treatment early because of adverse events. At a median follow-up of 97 months, there was no significant difference in the occurrence of contralateral breast cancer between the two groups. However further subgroup analysis showed that there was a possible benefit for premenopausal women in the treated group. They showed an adjusted HR = 0.66 (0.41–1.07) for developing contralateral breast cancer, and adjusted HR = 0.65 (0.46–0.92) for ipsilateral breast cancer. In postmenopausal women a reversal of this effect was seen with concomitant increases in the levels of new contralateral, HR = 1.32 (0.82–2.15), and ipsilateral breast cancer HR = 1.19 (0.75–1.89). There were no other significant effects observed. The rationale for this borderline significant effect is based on the interaction of fenretinide with insulin-like growth factor (IGF-I), lower levels of which are associated with a reduced risk of breast cancer. Fenretinide lowered levels of IGF-I in the treated premenopausal women but not in those who were postmenopausal. This observed effect, although interesting, requires further prospective analysis.

The results of this trial may lead to a chemoprevention study in young healthy women. There may also be a place for dual therapy studies with tamoxifen. This combination treatment has an enhanced effect in animal models.

Cyclo-oxygenase Inhibitors

There is a growing body of evidence that the inducible form of cyclo-oxygenase (COX) known as COX-2 is crucial for tumour angiogenesis[19]. In an *in vitro* model, Tsujii *et al.* observed that COX-2 positive colon cancer cells induced angiogenic changes in simultaneously cultured endothelial cells. The same investigators also reported that COX-2 positive tumour cell xenografts grew to significantly larger size compared with xenografts lacking COX-2. Furthermore, Swawaoka and colleagues observed that selective COX-2 inhibitors reduced the angiogenesis index and tumour growth of COX-2 positive carcinoma cells implanted in mice[20]. However, COX-2 inhibitors had no effect on angiogenesis or tumour growth of COX-2 negative carcinoma cells. The authors also suggested that COX-1 in the host endothelial cells may be required for a complete angiogenic response. Williams and colleagues used a combination implantation model and genetic engineering to address the relative role of host COX-1 and COX-2 in tumour angiogenesis[21]. The authors implanted COX-2 positive lung carcinoma cells in mice genetically engineered to lack either COX-1 or COX-2. Williams *et al.* observed a significant decrease in tumour growth and angiogenesis in COX-2 negative mice compared to COX-1 negative animals. Such observations support the current view that COX-2 expression in the host but in the tumour cells is required for tumour angiogenesis. Williams *et al.* also suggested that intracellular production of prostaglandin is required for the production of vascular endothelial growth factor (VEGF) by stromal cells since fibroblasts lacking COX-2 did not produce VEGF. However other researchers found that prostaglandins stimulated VEGF production in target cells[22]. The main difference between COX-1 and COX-2 is that the latter is easily inducible to high levels and, when stimulated, results in a significant increase in prostaglandins production. This may explain why COX-2 but not COX-1 is required for tumour growth and angiogenesis.

Animal experiments have shown that COX inhibitors can prevent or suppress cancer growth. COX-2 inhibition or knockout has been found to prevent adenomatous polyps development in mice carrying APC mutation[23]. Oshima *et al.* have also reported that COX-2 is over-expressed in the stromal cells of the colon rather than epithelial cells. In humans, COX-2 over-expression has been reported in various cancers[24,25]. Furthermore, epidemiological studies have shown that chronic intake of non-steroidal anti-inflammatory drugs (NSAIDs), which inhibit COX enzyme, significantly reduce the risk of colorectal cancer and polyps[26]. Harris *et al.*[27] observed that the selective COX-2 inhibitor celecoxib produced striking reductions in the incidence, multiplicity and volume of 7,12-dimethylbenz[α]anthracene (DMBA)-induced breast cancer in rats. Ibuprofen also produced significant effects but to a lesser extent. Hurang *et al.*[25] investigated COX-1 and COX-2 expression in human breast cancer specimens and reported over-expression of COX-2 in both primary tumours and stromal cells. COX-1 over-expression was primarily observed in stromal cells. Brueggemeier and colleagues[28] reported a significant correlation between COX and aromatase mRNA expressions in human breast cancer.

In a prospective cohort of 32 505 women followed up for 5 years, Harris and colleagues[29] found that regular intake of ibuprofen reduced breast cancer risk by 50% ($p < 0.01$). The risk was reduced by 40% in women regularly taking aspirin ($p < 0.05$). Such observations suggest that NSAIDs are likely to be effective chemopreventative agents against breast cancer.

Promising Molecular Target Agents

The complexity of ER targeting was increased by the recent discovery of ERβ. α and β receptors are genetically distinct and their interactions with SERMs reflect this. Tamoxifen has greater affinity for β and raloxifene for α receptors. The α : β ratio is different in breast cancer and normal breast tissue. Isoforms of the receptors also vary in breast cancer. Targeting molecular interactions downstream from ER receptors provides treatment strategies in the pharmacological management of ER-negative tumours, tamoxifen resistant tumours that are ER-positive (31%) and BRCA 1/2 carriers. The minutiae of the interaction between SERMs and estrogen receptors in these sub-groups remain to be unravelled.

Promising molecular target agents for breast cancer prevention include vitamin D analogues, polyamine biosynthesis inhibitors, arachidonic acid metabolizing enzyme (cyclo-oxygenase and lipo-oxygenase) inhibitors, telomerase inhibitors, cyclin dependant kinase inhibitors and retinoids. Gene therapy will only be applicable to the 0.7% of the population at risk (i.e. BRCA 1/2 carriers) but progress continues to offer hope to these women.

Conclusions

In conclusion there is a definite protective effect against breast cancer for women who take a low fat diet and exercise regularly. The SERMs may provide an effective method of chemoprevention if benefits seen in the NSABP trial can be maintained long term. Large randomized trials are required to assess the potential role of selective COX-2 inhibitors in chemoprevention. Fascinating research into other methods of prevention continues.

References

1. Freedman LS, Clifford C, Messina M. Analysis of dietary fat, calories, body weight and the development of mammary tumours in rats and mice, a review. *Cancer Res* 1990; **50**: 5710–5719.
2. Wu AH, Pike MC, Stam DO. Meta-analysis, dietary fat intake, serum estrogen levels and the risk of breast cancer. *J Natl Cancer Inst* 1999; **91**: 529–534.
3. Latikka P, Pukkala E, Vihko V. Relationship between the risk of breast cancer and physical activity: an epidemiological perspective (review). *Sports Med* 1998; **26**: 133–143.
4. Hilakivi-Clarke L, Onojafe I, Raygada M. Prepubertal exposure to zearalenone or genistein reduces mammary tumourigenesis. *Br J Cancer* 1999; **80**: 1682–1688.
5. Constantinou AI, Krygier AE, Mehta RR. Genistein induces maturation of cultured human breast cancer cells and prevents tumour growth in nude mice. *Am J Clin Nutrition* 1998; **68**: 1426S–1430S.
6. Key TJ, Sharp GB, Appleby PN *et al.* Soya foods and breast cancer risk, a prospective study in Hiroshima and Nagasaki, Japan. *Br J Cancer* 1999; **81**: 1248–1256.
7. Wu K, Helzlsouer KJ, Comstock GW *et al.* A prospective study on folate, B12 and pyridoxal 5'-phosphate (B6) and breast cancer. *Cancer Epidemiol Biomarkers Prev* 1999; **8**: 209–217.
8. Stoll BA. Western nutrition and the insulin resistance syndrome, a link to breast cancer. *Eur J Clin Nutr* 1999; **52**: 83–87.
9. Veronesi U, De Palo G, Marubini E *et al.* Randomised trial of fenretinide to prevent second breast malignancy in women with early stage breast cancer. *J Natl Cancer Inst* 1999; **91**: 1847–1856.
10. Lerner LJ, Jordan VC. Development of anti-estrogens and their use in breast cancer. Eighth Cain Memorial Lecture. *Cancer Res* 1990; **50**: 4177–4189.
11. Fisher B, Constantino JP, Wickerham DL *et al.* Tamoxifen for the prevention of breast cancer: report of the National Surgical Adjuvant Breast and Bowel Project P-1 Study. *J Natl Cancer Inst* 1998; **90**: 1371–1388.
12. Early Breast Cancer Trialists' Collaborative Group. Tamoxifen for early breast cancer: an overview of randomised trials. *Lancet* 1998; **351**: 1451–1462.
13. Powles T, Eeles R, Ashley S *et al.* Interim analysis of the incidence of breast cancer in the Royal Marsden Hospital tamoxifen randomised chemoprevention trial. *Lancet* 1998; **352**: 98–101.
14. Rebbeck TR, Levin AM, Eisen A *et al.* Breast cancer risk after bilateral prophylactic oophorectomy in BRCA1 mutation carriers. *J Natl Cancer Inst* 1999; **91**: 1475–1479.
15. Hatchlings O, Evans G, Fallowfield I *et al.* Effect of early American results in patients in the tamoxifen prevention trial. *Lancet* 1998; **352**: 1222 (letter).

16. Veronesi U, Maisonneuve P, Costa A *et al*. Prevention of breast cancer with tamoxifen, preliminary findings from the Italian randomised trial among hysterectomised women. *Lancet* 1998; **352**: 93–97.

17. Gail MH, Constantino JP, Bryant J *et al*. Weighing the risks and benefits of tamoxifen for preventing breast cancer. *J Natl Cancer Inst* 1999; **21**: 1829–1846.

18. Cummings SR, Eckert S, Kreuger *et al*. The effects of raloxifene on the risk of breast cancer in postmenopausal women. Results from the MORE randomised trial. *JAMA* 1999; **281**: 2189–2197.

19. Tsujii M, Kawano S, Tsuji S *et al*. Cyclo-oxygenase regulates angiogenesis induced by colon cancer cells. *Cell* 1998; **93**: 705–716.

20. Sawaoka H, Tsuji S, Tsujii M *et al*. Cyclo-oxygenase inhibitors suppress angiogenesis and reduce tumor growth in vivo. *Lab Invest* 1999; **79**: 1469–1477.

21. Williams CS, Tsujii M, Reese J *et al*. Host cyclo-oxygenase-2 modulates carcinoma growth. *J Clin Invest* 2000; **105**: 1589–1594.

22. Hoper MM *et al*. Prostaglandins induce vascular endothelial growth factor in a human monocytic cell line and rat lungs via cAMP. *Am J Respir Cell Mol Biol* 1997; **17**: 748–756.

23. Oshima M, Dinchuk JE, Kargman SL *et al*. Suppression of intestinal polyposis in Apc[716] knockout mice by inhibition of cyclooxygenase-2 (COX-2). *Cell* 1996; **87**: 803–809.

24. Prescott SM, Fitzpatrick FA. Cyclo-oxygenase-2 and carcinogenesis. *Biochim Biophys Acta* 2000; **1470**: M69–M78.

25. Hwang D, Scollard D, Byrne J *et al*. Expression of cyclo-oxygenase-1 and cyclo-oxygenase-2 in human breast cancer. *J Natl Cancer Inst* 1998; **90**: 455–466.

26. Giovannucci E, Egan KM, Hunter DJ *et al*. Aspirin and the risk of colorectal cancer in women. *N Engl J Med* 1995; **333**: 609–614.

27. Harris RE, Alshafie GA, Abou-Issa H *et al*. Chemoprevention of breast cancer in rats by celecoxib, a cyclo-oxygenase-2 inhibitor. *Cancer Res* 2000; **60**: 2101–2103.

28. Brueggemeier RW, Quinn AL, Parrett ML *et al*. Correlation of aromatase and cyclo-oxygenase gene expression in human breast cancer specimens. *Cancer Lett* 1999; **140**: 27–35.

29. Harris RE, Kasbari S, Farra WB. Prospective study of non-steroidal anti-inflammatory drugs and breast cancer. *Oncol Rep* 1999; **6**: 71–73.

10. Recent Advances in Biological Therapy

K. Mokbel

Introduction

The important discoveries in the field of molecular biology since the late 1980s and the integration of these research advances into clinical practice in the past few years have led to a 'biological war on cancer'. The recent advances in molecular biology therapy against breast cancer are concisely described and future directions are suggested. Important and promising molecular biological targets in the field of breast cancer include growth factor receptors, tyrosine kinases, angiogenesis, cyclo-oxygenase enzyme, oncogenes, telomerase enzyme and immunological processes.

Since such biological therapies are mainly cytostatic, it is likely that future drugs will require chronic administration in patients with early disease in order to prevent the growth of micrometastases. Molecular biological drugs are also likely to play a role in cancer prevention in high-risk patients. In advanced and metastatic disease, biological therapy is likely to be effective in combination with other treatments such as cytotoxic and hormonal drugs.

Antiangiogenesis Agents

The angiogenesis process seems to be essential for tumour growth beyond 1 mm[1]. Furthermore, the increase in tumour vascularization seems to increase the risk of distant metastases[2]. Angiogenesis arises as a result of altered equilibrium between positive and negative regulators[3]. Factors involved in angiogenesis include: vascular endothelial growth factor (VEGF), fibroblastic growth factor (FGF), platelet-derived growth factor (PDGF), interleukin 8 (IL-8), interferon beta (INF-β), platelet-derived endothelial cell growth factor (PD-ECGF), tumour-necrosis factors alpha (TNF-α), thrombospondin, transforming growth factor alpha and beta (TGF-α and β) and hepatocyte growth factor (HGF). Increased VEGF expression (mRNA or protein) was found to be associated with increased microvessel density and poor clinical outcome in patients with breast cancer[5].

Therapeutic strategies that interfere with angiogenesis currently in development include inhibition of angiogenesis receptor-related tyrosine kinases[6], inhibition of matrix metalloproteinases, interferon administration, inhibition of cyclo-oxygenase-2 (COX-2) enzyme[7] and blockade of epidermal growth factor receptor (EGFR)[8].

Inhibitors of COX-2 and EGFR are discussed in subsequent sections of this chapter. Since angiogenesis in healthy adults is restricted to wound healing, pregnancy and corpus luteum formation, angiogenesis inhibitors potentially have therefore a wide therapeutic window.

Flk-1/KDR Inhibitors

In 1998, Sun *et al.*[9] reported the synthesis of a novel synthetic tyrosine kinase (TK) inhibitor by substituting the R1 and R2 positions of the inolin-2-one structure. Several such compounds were subsequently synthesized with different inhibitory profiles to tyrosine kinase proteins. One compound synthesized by Sugen known as SU5416 (Figure 1) has been found to be a more potent inhibitor than other structurally related compounds and has therefore entered clinical trials. *In vitro* studies showed that SU5416 was a potent inhibitor of VEGR-TK and PDGFR-TK but a weak inhibitor of GFR-TK. The signalling transduction activity of both VEGR type 1 (Flt-1) and type 2 (Flk-1/KDR) seems to be inhibited by SU5416[10]. Subsequently, *in vivo* studies demonstrated a

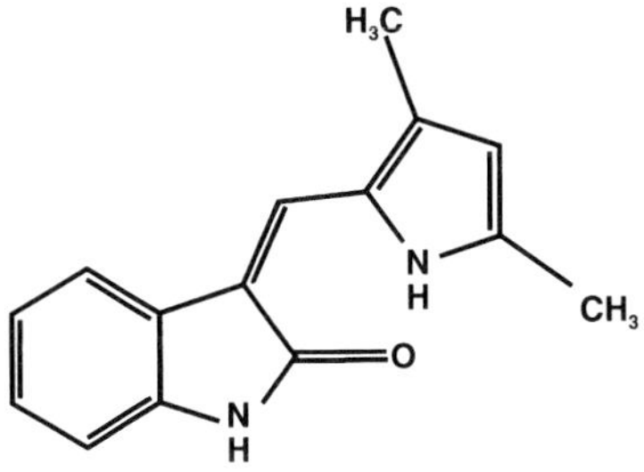

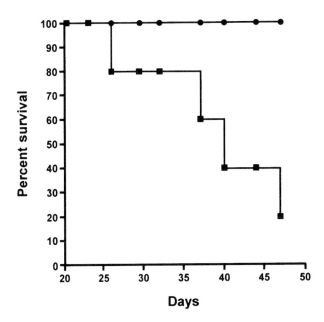

Figure 1 Structure of SU5416

significant inhibition by SU5416 of the growth of several types of subcu-taneous xenografts in mice (Figure 2)[6,11]. SU5416 was the first com-pound with inolin-2-one core structure to enter clinical trials. The first patient was treated in 1997. In a phase 1 study, 69 patients with advanced cancers were treated using SU5416 with good tolerability and minimal toxicity[12]. Phase III clinical trials in colorectal cancer and

Figure 2 Survival curve for tumour-bearing mice treated with SU5416, 25 mg/kg/day (circles) or DMSO (squares) as a control. All mice were initially treated with cyclophosphamide (200 mg/kg) as a control. Adapted from Mendel *et al. Anticancer Drug Design*, 2000; **15**: 29–41

NSCCL are currently underway. The recommended dose is 145 mg/m^2 s.c. twice weekly. The evidence suggests that SU5416 is an effective cytostatic drug against solid tumours and clinical trials using the drug in breast cancer are expected to commence soon.

Two other small molecules capable of inhibiting Flk-1/KDR are currently being developed. ZD4190, being developed by AstraZeneca, can inhibit VEGFR-TK, VEGF-stimulated human umbilical vein endothelial cells (HUVEC) proliferation in culture and tumour growth in xenograft models and vascular permeability. The other compound, known as CGP 79787, has been observed to prolong survival and reduce ascites in human ovarian cancer xenograft animal model. This drug is being developed by Novartis. Both agents are currently in phase I clinical trials. In view of the cytostatic activity of these small molecules, it is likely that they will be used in combination with other drugs such as cytotoxic agents and will be effective in the treatment of locally advanced and metastatic breast cancer.

Other Inhibitors of Angiogenesis Gowth Factors

Sugen has also developed SU6668 which has entered phase I clinical trials. The drug inhibits receptor tyrosine kinases involved in the angiogenesis process, tumour cell proliferation and endothelial cell growth and migration[13]. SU6668 has been shown to be effective against several tumour xenograft models.

The recombinant humanized monoclonal anti-VEGF antibody developed by Genentech has recently entered phase II and III clinical trials on breast cancer.

Other antiangiogenic agents that inhibit VEGF function include Angiozyme (Ribozyme Pharmaceuticals) and RTK787 (Novartis). The former inactivates mRNA of two VEGF receptors and the latter inhibits phosphorylation which is required for the signal transduction by VEGF and PDGF receptors.

Matrix Metalloproteinases (MMPs) Inhibitors

MMPs have been selected as targets for anticancer therapy in view of their important role in tumour angiogenesis and invasion. Agouron

Pharmaceuticals have developed AG3340 which is a potent inhibitor of MMPs, 2, 9, 13 and 14. The drug was shown to effectively inhibit the growth of several tumour xenograft models including breast carcinoma[14]. The efficacy of the compound was enhanced by combining it with cytotoxic agents1[5]. Such a combination was found to be well-tolerated in phase I clinical trials. Phase III clinical trials in non-squamous cell carcinoma of the lung (NSCLC) and hormone-refractory prostate cancer are currently in progress.

Marimastat is a less selective MMP inhibitor which has been developed by British Biotech. This drug is orally bioavailable and its main side-effects include fatigue and dose-dependent polyarthritis. Marimastat has been shown to be effective in the treatment of inoperable gastric and pancreatic cancer and phase III clinical trials in breast, colon, ovarian and lung cancer are ongoing[16].

Bay12-9566 is another orally-active MMP inhibitor. The drug selectively inhibits MMP-2 and MMP-9. Although it lacks significant musculoskeletal toxicity, it has been reported to cause dose-dependent hepatic toxicity and bone marrow toxicity. Preliminary observations from phase III studies have suggested a detrimental effect on survival and therefore the drug has been withdrawn[16].

Neovastat is an oral MMP inhibitor which has been extracted from shark cartilage. The drug has entered phase III clinical trials in NSCLC and colorectal cancer[16]. Other MMP inhibitors in development (phase I/II) include Solimastat (BB2516), COL-3, BMS-275291 and CGS27023A.

Interferon-alpha (INF-α)

The INF family includes three types of glycoproteins: INF-α which is derived from leukocytes, INF-β which is derived from fibroblasts and INF-γ which is derived from immunocytes. INFs seem to exert their antiangiogenic effects by inhibiting FGF and endothelial cell growth factor (ECGF) induced endothelial cell proliferation[17,18], the motility of endothelial cells[19] and the expression of metalloproteinases[20]. The antiangiogenic effects of INFs seem to be independent of their antiproliferative effects. INF-α has been widely used in the treatment of human tumours including melanoma, renal cell carcinoma and transitional cell carcinoma with limited response. However, this cytokine has been found more effective in the treatment of Kaposi's sarcoma in view of its antiangiogenic properties[21]. Furthermore, transfection with the mRNA-beta has been recently investigated in the treatment of human cancer in preclinical xenograft tumour models[22]. The role of INFs in the treatment of breast cancer in combination with other treatment modality is currently under investigation.

Other Angiogenesis Inhibitors[16]

Inhibitors of Endothelial Cell Activation

Such drugs include TNP-470 (TAP Pharmaceuticals), Squalamine (Magainin) and Endostatin (Entremed). TNP-470 and Squalamine are currently in phase II clinical trials.

Agents Targeting Tumour Vasculature

Vitaxin (Ixsys) and EMD121974 (Merck) target integrins present in tumour vasculature. Both drugs have recently entered phase II clinical trials.

CM101 (AstraZeneca) and Combrestatin (Oxigen) are still at the phase I clinical trial stage.

Miscellaneous

Several agents seem to inhibit angiogenesis via multiple or unknown mechanisms. Such agents include thalidomide, IM862, suramin and analogues, penicillamine, interleukin-12, captopril, taxanes and razoxane.

References

1. Folkman J. Angiogenesis in cancer, vascular, rheumatoid and other disease. *Nature Med* 1995; **1**: 27–31.
2. Fontanini G, Bigini D, Vignati S *et al.* Microvessel count predicts metastatic disease and survival in non small cell lung cancer. *J Pathol* 1995; **177**: 57.

3. Liotta LA, Steeg PS, Stetlet-Stevenson WG. Cancer metastasis and angiogenesis: an imbalance of positive and negative regulation. *Cell* 1991; **4**: 327–336.

4. Fiddler IJ. Angiogenesis and cancer metastasis. *Cancer J* 2000; **6**: S134–S141.

5. Scott PA, Smith K, Poulson R *et al*. *Br J Cancer* 1998; **77**: 2120–2128.

6. Mendel DB, Laird D, Smolich DB *et al*. Development of SU5416, a selective small molecule inhibitor of VEGF receptor tyrosine kinase activity as an antiangiogenesis agent. *Anti-Cancer Drug Design* 2000; **15**: 29–41.

7. Masferrer J, Zwerfel S, Heuvelman M *et al*. COX-2 inhibition of angiogenesis suppresses tumour growth in tumours that either express cyclo-oxygenases or do not. *Proc Am Assoc Cancer Res* 2000; **646**: Abstr. 4106.

8. Cullinane C, Kleinschmidt M, Webster LK. Antitumour activity of ZD1839 (Iressa) in combination with Cisplatin in NIH3T3 cells expressing epidermal growth factor receptor. *Proc Am Assoc Cancer Res* 2000: Abstr 3073.

9. Sun L, Tran N. Tang F *et al*. Synthesis and biological evaluations of 3-substituted indolin-2-ones: a novel class of tyrosine kinase inhibitors that exhibit selectivity towards particular receptor tyrosine kinases. *J Med Chem* 1998; **41**: 2588–2603.

10. Armesilla AL, Lorenzo E, Gomez del Arco P *et al*. Vascular endothelial growth factor activates nuclear factor of activated T-cells in human endothelial cells: a role for tissue factor gene expression. *Mol Cell Biol* 1999; **19**: 2032–2043.

11. Fong TA, Shawver LK, Sun L *et al*. SU5416 is a potent and selective inhibitor of the vascular endothelial growth factor receptor (Flk-1/KDR) that inhibits tyrosine kinase catalysis, tumour vascularisation and growth of multiple cancer types. *Cancer Res* 1999; **59**: 99–106.

12. Rosen L, Mulay M, Mayers A *et al*. Phase I dose-escalating trial of SU5416, a novel angiogenesis inhibitor in patients with advanced malignancies. *Proceedings of the 35th Annual Meeting of the American Society of Clinical Oncology* 1999, Atlanta GA, Abstract 618.

13. Klohs WD, Hamdy JM. Antiangiogenic agents. *Curr Opin Biotechnol* 1999; **10**: 544–549.

14. Shalinsky DR, Brekken J, Zou H *et al*. Broad antitumour and antiangiogenic activities of AG3340, a potent and selective MMP inhibitor undergoing advanced oncology clinical trials. *Ann Y Acad Sci* 1999; **878**: 236–270.

15. Shalinsky DR, Brekken J, Zou H *et al*. Marked antiangiogenic and antitumourefficacy of AG3340 in chemoresistant human non-small cell lung cancer tumours: single agent and combination chemotherapy studies. *Clin Cancer Res* 1999; **5**: 1905–1917.

16. Daplanque G, Harris AL. Anti-angiogenic agents: clinical trial design and therapies in development. *Eur J Cancer* 2000; **36**: 1713–1724.

17. Heyns AP, Eldor A, Vlodavsky I *et al.* The antiproliferative effect of interferon and the mitogenic activity of growth factors are independent cell cycle events. *Exp Cell Res* 1985; **161**: 297–306.
18. Friesel R, Komoriya A, Maciag T. Inhibition of endothelial cell proliferation by gamma-interferon. *J Cell Biol* 1987; **104**: 1689–696.
19. Brouty-Boye D, Zetter BR. Inhibition of cell motility by interferon. *Science* 1988; **208**: 516–518.
20. Kato N, Nawa A, Tamakoshi K *et al.* Suppression of gelatines, production with decreased invasiveness of choriocarcinoma cells by human recombinant interferon beta. *Am J Obstet Gynecol* 1995; **172**: 601–606.
21. Mitsuyasu RT. Interferon-alpha in the treatment of AIDS-related Kaposi's sarcoma. *Br J Haematol* 1991; **79**: 69–73.
22. Dong Z, Greene G, Pettaway C *et al.* Suppression of angiogenesis, tumorigenicity and metastasis by human prostate cancer cells, engineered to produce interferon-beta. *Cancer Res* 1999; **59**: 872–879.

EGFR Tyrosine Kinase Inhibitors

Epidermal growth factor receptor (EGFR) is a 170-kilodalton transmembrane glycoprotein, the phosphorylation of which after dimerization leads to cellular activation of mitogenic transduction signals[1]. EGFR is over-expressed in a wide range of human cancers including breast cancer. Over-expression of EGFR is linked to a more aggressive tumour behaviour, poorer clinical outcome and resistance to chemotherapy[2]. Therefore, drugs that block EGFR have a potential in treating patients with breast cancer and increasing sensitivity to chemo-therapy in patients with chemoresistant tumours. ZD1839 (Iressa, AstraZeneca®) is an orally active selective inhibitor of EGFR tyrosine kinase, which has been shown to inhibit the growth of EGFR expressing human breast cancer cell line (HER 14) in a dose-dependent fashion[3] and decrease the proliferation index and increase the apoptotic index of DCIS xenografts[4]. Furthermore, ZD 1839 has increased the chemo-sensitivity to cisplatin in HER 14 cells lines[3].

Phase 1 studies have demonstrated that Iressa is efficacious and well tolerated when administered orally in patients with solid tumours, par-ticularly in patients with non-squamous cell carcinoma of the lung (NSCLC)[5,6]. The structure of ZD1839 is shown in Figure 3.

Preclinical studies have demonstrated that PD 0169414 can irrevers-ibly inhibit EGFR family tyrosine kinases with low IC_{50} values[7]. The oral administration of PD 0169414 has been shown to reduce tyrosine phosphorylation on the EGFR and inhibit tumour growth in A431 tumour xenografts. The drug has recently entered phase I clinical trials.

Pfizer have recently developed an EGFR inhibitor (CP-358,774) with similar properties to ZD1839 and PD 0169414. The drug was found to be well tolerated in phase I clinical trials[8].

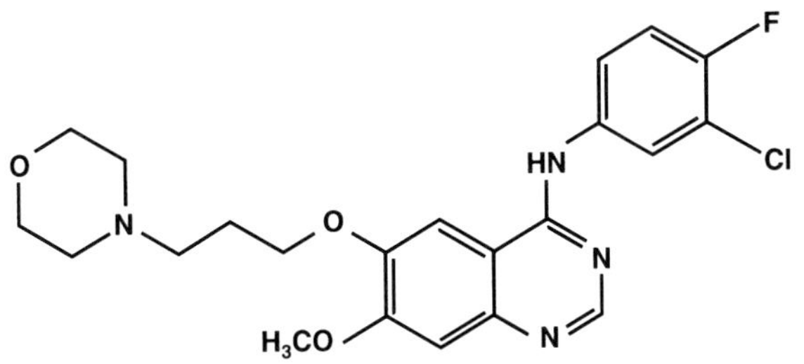

Figure 3   Structure of ZD1839

EGFR antibodies in cancer therapy has also been investigated. A monoclonal antibody (mAb225) against EGFR has been shown to competitively inhibit EGF binding at block activation of EGFR-TK. Win *et al.* demonstrated that mAb225 inhibited the growth of a human colorectal cancer cell line (DiFi) that expresses a high level of EGFR and encouraged the cells to enter apoptosis[8]. The compound seems to enhance the tumour response to cytotoxic agents and radiotherapy, and therefore phase II and III trials of C225 in combination with chemotherapy and/or radiotherapy are currently in progress.

References

1. Woodburn J. The epidermal growth factor receptor and its inhibition in cancer therapy. *Pharmacol Ther* 1999; **82**: 241–250.
2. Ciardiello F, Bianco R, Damiano V *et al.* Antitumour activity of sequential treatment with topotecan and anti-epidermal growth factor receptor monoclonal antibody C225. *Clin Cancer Res* 1999; **5**: 909–916.
3. Cullinane C, Kleinschmidt M, Webster LK. Anti-tumour activity of ZD 1839 (Iressa) in combination with cisplatin in NIH 3T3 cells expressing human epidermal growth factor receptor. *Proc Am Assoc Cancer Res* 2000; Abstr. 3073.
4. Chan KC, Gandhi A, Knox WF *et al.* ZD1839 (Iressa), an epidermal growth factor receptor for tyrosine kinase inhibitor, decreases epithelial proliferation in DCIS of the breast, whereas C-erbB2 monoclonal antibody (Trastuzumab) blockade does not. *Proc Am Assoc Cancer Res* 2000; Abstr. 3074.
5. Ferry D, Hammond L, Ranson M *et al.* Intermittent oral ZD1839(Iressa), a novel epidermal growth factor receptor tyrosine kinase inhibitor (EGFR-TKI), shows evidence of good tolerability and activity: final results from a phase I study. *Proc Am Soc Clin Oncol* 2000; Abstr. 5E.
6. Baselga J, Herbst R, Lorusso P *et al.* Continuing administration of ZD1839 (Iressa), a novel epidermal growth factor receptor. Tyrosine kinase inhibitor (EGFR-TKI) in patients with five selected tumour types: evidence of activity and good tolerability. *Proc Am Soc Clin Oncol* 2000; Abstr. 686.
7. Vincent PW, Bridges AJ, Dykes DJ *et al.* Anticancer efficacy of the irreversible EGFr tyrosine kinase inhibitor PD 0169414 against human tumour xenografts. *Cancer Chemother Pharmacol* 2000; **45**: 231–238.
8. Wu X, Fan Z, Masui H *et al.* Apoptosis induced by an anti-epidermal growth factor receptor monoclonal antibody in human colorectal carcinoma cell line and its delay by insulin. *J Clin Invest* 1995; **95**: 1897–1905.

Immunotherapy

Immunotherapy is a relatively new approach to cancer management. Although this approach has been extensively investigated in some solid tumours such as renal cell carcinoma and melanoma, its role in the management of breast cancer has not been adequately investigated.

Immunotherapeutic approaches include cytokine administration (e.g. INFs), monoclonal antibodies against tumour antigens (e.g. Herceptin), tumour vaccines using tumour associated antigens (TAAs), T-cell therapy and immunotoxins. The recent observation that a natural humoral immune response to polymorphic epithelial mucin (MUC1) predicts for a favourable outcome in women with early breast cancer supports the hypothesis that immunization with MUC1 as an antigen may have a potential in breast cancer therapy[1]. HER-2 protein has also been used as a target for immunization. In an animal model, Amici *et al.* demonstrated the effectiveness of DNA vaccination using truncated new plasmins in inducing antitumour protection[2]. Matory *et al.* observed significant antitumour effects after INF-α gene transfection in a mouse breast cancer model[3]. Several authors have observed antitumour activity of IL-10 expressed as a transgene or administered as a recombinant protein.

Recent evidence suggests that nitric oxide and INF-gamma play an important role in tumour immunotherapy with IL-10[4]. More recently, a phase 1 clinical trial examining the role of TALL-104 cells in patients with resistant metastatic breast cancer has been carried out[5]. TALL-104 is a human cytotoxic T-cell line. The results of this study demonstrated good tolerability by patients and warranted further research in the field. The role of dendritic cells is also being investigated.

References

1. Von-Mensdorff-Pouilly S, Verstraeten AA, Kenemans P *et al.* Survival in early breast cancer patients is favourably influenced by a natural humoral immune response to polymorphic epithelial mucin. *J Clin Oncol* 2000; **18**: 574–583.
2. Amici A, Smorlesi A, Noce G *et al.* DNA vaccination with full-length or truncated neu induces protective immunity against the development of spontaneous mammary tumours in HER-2/neu transgenic mice. *Gene Ther* 2000; **7**: 703–706.

3. Matory YL, Dorfman DM, Wu L. Treatment of established tumour is associated with ICAM-1 upregulation and reversed by CD8 depletion in a tumour necrosis factor-alpha gene transfected mouse mammary tumour. *Pathobiology* 1999; **67**: 186–195.
4. Sun H, Guttierrez P, Jackson MJ *et al.* Essential role of nitric oxide and interferon-gamma for tumour immunotherapy with interleukin-10. *J Immunother* 2000; **23**: 208–214.
5. Visonneau S, Cesano A, Porter DL. Phase I trial of TALL-104 cells in patients with refractory metastatic breast cancer. *Clin Cancer Res* 2000; **695**:1744–1754.

Anti-HER-2 Antibody (Herceptin)

Introduction

The HER-2/neu proto-oncogene (also known as c-erbB-2) was first described in 1984 by Schechter *et al.*[1]. The gene encodes a 185-kilodalton transmembrane glycoprotein with intrinsic tyrosine kinase activity. The protein also exhibits extensive homology to epidermal growth factor receptor (EGFR)[2,3]. HER-2 over-expression occurs in 25–30% of breast carcinomas and was found to be a poor prognostic factor in both node-negative and node-positive invasive carcinomas[4,5] and ductal carcinoma *in situ*[6]. Furthermore, HER-2 over-expression was found to predict better response to doxorubicin[7] and worse response to hormonal therapy[8]. Preclinical studies using a monoclonal antibody against HER-2 oncoprotein showed anti-breast cancer activity and suggested an antiangiogenic as well as an immunogenic mechanism of action[9,10].

Clinical Efficacy and HER-2 Testing

A recent phase III multicentre randomized clinical trial has shown that the addition of Herceptin (a recombinant humanized IgG$_1$ monoclonal antibody against HER-2) to first-line chemotherapy (e.g. Paclitaxel) significantly prolongs the time to tumour progression (TTP) and produces a greater objective response in patients with HER-2 over-expressing metastatic breast cancer[11] (Table 1). In another phase III trial, Herceptin (trastuzumab) as a single agent was found to be efficacious and safe in 222 women with HER-2 over-expressing metastatic breast cancer that had relapsed after chemotherapy[12]. HER-2 expression in breast cancer can be determined by measuring mRNA expression using the FISH technique (fluorescent in situ hybridization) or using immunohistochemical methods. However, immunohistochemistry does not always correlate well with the former. In a recent study examining the sensitivity of three frequently used HER-2 antibodies in archival tissue samples of invasive breast cancer, it was observed that the monoclonal antibody raised against the external domain (TAB250) had the lowest misclassification rate (9.6%) of HER-2 expression as determined by

Table 1 **Herceptin efficacy in HER-2 overexpressing patients (3+ score by IHC)**

Parameter	H + P n = 68	P n = 77	H n = 172
Median duration of response (months)	8.3	4.6	9.1
Median survival (months)	24.8	17.9	16.4
Median TTP (months)	7.1	3.0	3.2
Response rates (%)	49	17	18

IHC, immunohistochemistry; H, Herceptin; P, Paclitaxel; TTP, time to progression

FISH techniques[13]. It is currently recommended that HER-2 status is initially determined immunohistochemically using the HercepTest and a standard scoring system (0, 1+, 2+, or 3+). Patients with tumours showing 3+ are considered eligible for Herceptin treatment. Tumours showing 2+ should be tested by FISH and if the latter is positive then the patient is considered eligible for Herceptin therapy (Table 2).

The encouraging results of trastuzumab in women with HER-2 over-expressing metastatic breast cancer have led researchers to investigate the role of trastuzumab–chemotherapy combination as a means of improving response rates. Two presentations at the 22nd Annual San Antonio Breast Cancer Symposium (1999) addressed this issue. Winer and colleagues observed overall response in 24 (71%) of 34 women with HER-2 over-expressing metastatic breast cancer when treated with Herceptin and vinorelbine. Furthermore, the authors observed few serious toxicities. Dr Estera from the University of Texas Houston Medical School also reported a 74% response rate (>50% reduction in size) in 63 women with metastatic breast cancer positive for HER-2 expression as determined by monoclonal (TAB 250 and CB11) and polyclonal (HercepTest and PAB1) antibodies.

Table 2   The recommended immunohistochemistry scoring system of HER-2 expression

Staining pattern	Score	HER-2 status
No staining observed	0	Negative
Membrane staining in less than 10% of tumour cells	0	Negative
Barely perceptible membrane staining in >10% of tumour cells	1+	Negative
Faint staining of part of the membrane of >10% of tumour cells	1+	Negative
Weak to moderate complete membrane staining of >10% of tumour cells	2+	Weak to moderate over-expression
Moderate to strong complete membrane staining of >10% of tumour cells	3+	Moderate to strong over-expression

N.B. Only patients with tumour scoring 3+ are considered eligible for Herceptin therapy. FISH testing is recommended for tumours scoring 2+ and if FISH is positive then Herceptin should be considered.

Dose and Administration

Herceptin is administered as a 90-minute infusion (2 mg/kg) once weekly after an initial loading dose (4 mg/kg). The patient should be observed for 2 hours after administration to monitor for infusion-related reactions. The treatment should be continued until disease progression. However the issue of treatment duration has not been adequately addressed by the clinical trials thus far.

Adverse Effects and Contraindications

Herceptin is relatively well tolerated when compared with cytotoxic chemotherapy. The most common adverse reactions are infusion-related symptoms such as fever and chills, usually after the first administration. Adverse effects occurring in more than 10% of patients in the two pivotal clinical trials include: abdominal pain, diarrhoea, headaches, arthralgia, chest pain, chills, myalgia and rash. Serious pulmonary events and haematological toxicity have been infrequently reported. Symptomatic cardiac failure has been observed in approximately 8.5% and hepatic toxicity has occurred in 12% of patients.

The contraindications to Herceptin therapy include hypersensitivity to trastuzumab or murine proteins and severe dyspnoea at rest requiring oxygen therapy.

Future Directions

The role of serum levels of the extracellular domain (ECD, P105) in predicting and monitoring response to therapy requires further evaluation and clarification.

Future trials may demonstrate Herceptin efficacy in the adjuvant setting thus improving further the survival of some patients with early breast cancer.

References

1. Schechter AL, Stern DF, Vaidyanathan L *et al*. The neu oncogene: an erb-B related gene encoding a 185 000-M tumour antigen. *Nature* 1984; **312**: 513–516.
2. Akiyama T, Sudo C, Ogawara H *et al*. The product of the human c-erbB-2 gene: a 185-kilodalton glycoprotein with tyrosine kinase activity. *Science* 1986; **232**: 1644–1646.
3. Coussens L, Yang-Feng TL, Laio YC *et al*. Tyrosine kinase receptor with extensive homology to EGF receptor shares chromosomal location with neu oncogene. *Science* 1985; **230**: 1132–1139.
4. Slamon DJ, Clark GM, Wong SG *et al*. Human breast cancer correlation of relapse and survival with amplification of the HER/2 neu oncogene. *Science* 1987; **235**: 177–182.
5. Andrullis IL, Bull SB, Blackstein ME *et al*. Neu/erbB-2 amplification identifies a poor prognosis group of women with node-negative breast cancer. *J Clin Oncol* 1998; **16**: 1340–1349.
6. Evans A, Pinder S, Wilson R *et al*. Ductal carcinoma in situ of the breast: correlation between mammographic and pathologic findings. *AJR* 1994; **162**: 1307–1311.

7. Paik S, Bryant J, Park C *et al.* ErbB-2 and response to doxorubicin in patients with axillary lymph node-positive hormone receptor-negative breast cancer. *J Natl Cancer Inst* 1998; **90**: 1361-1370.

8. Bianco AR, De Laurentis M, Carlomagno C *et al.* Her-2 over-expression predicts adjuvant tamoxifen failure for early breast cancer: complete data at 20 years of the Naples GUN randomised trial. *Proc Am Soc Clin Oncol* 2000; **75a**: Abstr 289.

9. Hudziak RM, Lewis GD, Winget M *et al.* A p185 [HER2] monoclonal antibody has antiproliferative effects in vitro and sensitises human breast tumour cells to tumour necrosis factor. *Mol Cell Biol* 1989; **9**: 1165–1172.

10. Petit AM, Rak J, Hung MC *et al.* Neutralizing antibodies against epidermal growth factor and erbB-2/neu receptor tyrosine kinase down-regulate vascular endothelial growth factor production by tumour cells in vitro and in vivo: angiogenic implications for signal transduction of solid tumours. *Am J Pathol* 1997; **151**: 1523–1530.

11. Slamon D, Leyland-Jones B, Shak S *et al.* Addition of Herceptin[TM] (humanised Anti-HER-2 antibody) to first line chemotherapy for HER-2 overexpressing metastatic breast cancer (HER-2+/-MBC) markedly increases anticancer activity:a randomised multinational controlled phase III trial. *Proc Am Soc Clin Oncol* 1998; Abstr 377.

12. Cobleigh MA, Vogel CL, Tripathy D *et al.* Efficacy and safety of Herceptin[TM] (humanized Anti-HER-2 antibody) as a single agent in 222 women with HER2 overexpression who relapsed following chemotherapy for metastatic breast cancer. *Proc Am Soc Clin Oncol* 1998; Abstr 376.

13. Gancberg D, Lespagnard L, Rouas G *et al.* Sensitivity of HER-2/neu antibodies in archival tissue samples of invasive breast carcinomas. Correlation with oncogene amplification in 160 cases. *Am J Clin Pathol* 2000; **113**: 675–682.

Bisphosphonates

Osteolytic bone metastases are relatively common in patients with breast cancer. Osteolytic bone lesions may cause bone pain, pathological fractures and spinal cord compression. Surgical intervention or radiotherapy may be required to treat or prevent such skeletal complications. Bone destruction seems to be caused by osteoclast stimulation and its response to hormonal and/or chemotherapy has been limited.

Bisphosphonates such as pamidronates and clodronates are potent inhibitors of osteoclasts and have the potential of treating osteolytic bone metastases and preventing their complications.

Follow-up results from two prospective multicentre randomized double-blind placebo-controlled intervention trials have demonstrated that pamidronate infusion (90 mg monthly) is well tolerated and superior to antineoplastic therapy alone in preventing skeletal complications (51 vs 64%, $p < 0.001$) and palliating symptoms in women with stage IV breast cancer and osteolytic bone metastases for at least 24 months[1]. Furthermore, Diel et al. observed that oral bisphosphonates significantly reduced the number of bone metastases and possibly visceral metastases in women with breast cancer. The authors have recently reported the results of extended follow-up duration (median follow-up = 53 months). A total of 302 women with breast cancer associated with bone marrow micrometastases were randomized to oral clodronate (1600 mg daily) for 2 years or simply followed-up[2]. Oral clodronate has significantly reduced the incidence of bone metastases ($p = 0.044$) but the reduction in visceral metastases has failed to reach statistical significance ($p = 0.09$). However, the effect of clodronate after extended follow-up has been much weakened. Zoledronate is a new generation bisphosphonate that has been shown to be superior to pamidronate in the treatment of malignant hypercalcaemia[3].

In vitro studies have demonstrated that bisphosphonates induce apoptosis in breast cancer cell lines (MCF7 and MDA231) and may enhance response rates when combined with cytotoxic or hormonal therapy[4]. Such effects can be investigated in vivo by determining apoptosis of micrometastases in the bone marrow of breast cancer patients. Further clinical trials with large numbers and longer follow-up are required in order to assess the role of bisphosphonates in reducing the incidence of skeletal complications and visceral metastases in women with early and advanced breast cancer. The mechanism of action of these agents and potential interactions with growth factors and cytokines are worth investigating.

References

1. Lipton A, Theriault R, Hortobaggi G *et al.* Pamidronate prevents skeletal complications and is an effective palliative treatment in women with breast carcinoma and osteolytic bone metastases. *Cancer* 2000; **88**: 1082–1090.
2. Gollan C, Schutz F, Bastert G *et al.* Bisphosphonate in the reduction of metastases in breast cancer: results of the extended follow-up of the first study population. *Proc Am Soc Clin Oncol* 2000; **82A**: Abstr. 314.
3. Major B, Lortholany A, Hon J *et al.* Zoledronic acid is superior to pamidronate in the treatment of tumour-induced hypercalcaemia: a pooled analysis. *Proc Am Soc Clin Oncol* 2000; **605a**: Abstr. 2382.
4. Jagder SP, Croucher PI, Coleman RE. Zoledronate induces apoptosis of breast cancer cells. In vitro evidence for additive and synergistic effects with Taxol and tamoxifen. *Proc Am Soc Clin Oncol* 2000; **664a**: Abstr. 2619.

COX-2 Inhibitors

Cyclo-oxygenase-2 (COX-2) represents the inducible form of the COX system and has been found to be associated with carcinogenesis and to be upregulated in breast cancer[1]. COX-2 expression is also upregulated in new blood vessels of tumours suggesting that COX-2 products play an important role in angiogenesis[2].

Observational studies demonstrated a protective effect for NSAIDs against colorectal cancer[3]. In a small prospective trial, sulindac was found to decrease the number of polyps by 44% in patients with FAP4. COX-2 expression has been detected in 45% of pre-malignant adenomas and 85% of colorectal carcinomas. This observation, in addition to preclinical studies, suggest that COX-2 acts as a promoter of carcinogenesis[1].

Recent evidence suggests that selective COX-2 inhibitors such as celecoxib can inhibit growth and angiogenesis of COX-positive and COX-negative cell lines (HT-29 and HCT-116 respectively) by approximately 50%[5]. More recent studies have shown that COX-2 inhibitors increase the sensitivity of malignant cells to radiotherapy and chemotherapy[6]. Clinical trials examining the role of COX-2 inhibitors in the treatment and prevention of breast cancer are required.

References

1. How LR, Subaramaiah K, Chung WJ *et al.* Transcriptional activation of cyclo-oxygenase-2 in Wnt-1 transformed mammary epithelial cells. *Cancer Res* 1999; **59**: 1572–1577.
2. Jones MK, Wang H, Peskar BM *et al.* Inhibition of angiogenesis by nonsteroidal anti-inflammatory drugs: insight into mechanisms and implications for cancer growth and ulcer healing. *Nature Med* 1999; **5**: 1418–1423.
3. Giovannucci E, Egan KM, Hunter DJ *et al.* Aspirin and the risk of colorectal cancer in women. *N Engl J Med* 1995; **333**: 609–614.
4. Giardiello M, Hamilton SR, Krush AJ *et al.* Treatment of colonic and rectal adenomas with sulindac in familial adenomatous polyposis. *N Engl J Med* 1993; **328**: 1313–1316.
5. Masferrer J, Zweifel BS, Heuvelman M *et al.* COX-2 inhibitors of angiogenesis suppresses tumour growth in tumours that either express cycloxygensases or do not. *Proc Am Assoc Cancer Res* 2000; **646**: Abstr. 4106
6. More J, Zweifel BS, Heuvelman M *et al.* Enhanced antitumour activity by co-administration of celecoxib and the chemotherapeutic agents cyclophosphamide and 5-FU. *Proc Am Assoc Cancer Res* 2000; **409**: Abstr. 2600.

Farnesyl Transferase Inhibitors

The post-translational addition of a farnesyl moiety to the ras oncoprotein is essential for its membrane localization and biological activity in malignant transformation. Therefore, farnesyl transferase is a potential target for anticancer therapy in patients with ras-dependent tumours. XR3054, which is structurally similar to farnesyl, has been shown to reduce the farnesylation of p21 in a dose-dependent fashion[1]. L-744,832, another selective inhibitor of farnesyl transferase, was observed to induce irreversible regression of mammary tumours in mice[2]. R11577 is another farnesyl transferase inhibitor which is active orally. The results of a phase II trial in 27 patients with advanced breast cancer were presented at the recent ASCO meeting[3]. Three (12%) patients had a 'partial response and a further nine patients (35%) had a stable disease after 3 months of treatment. Myelotoxicity was the most frequent adverse effect and dose-limiting factor. Further studies examining the role of farnesyl transferase inhibitors are required.

References

1. Donaldson MJ, Skoumas V, Watson M *et al.* XR3054, structurally related to limonene, is a novel inhibitor of farnesyl protein transferase. *Eur J Cancer* 1999; **35**: 1014–1019.
2. Norgaard P, Law B, Joseph H *et al.* Treatment with farnesyl-protein transferase inhibitor induces regression of mammary tumours in transforming growth factor (TGF) alpha and TGF alpha/neu transgenic mice by inhibition of mitogenic activity and induction of apoptosis. *Clin Cancer Res* 1999; **5**: 35–42.
3. Johnston SR, Ellis PA Houston S *et al.* A phase II study of the farnesyl transferase inhibitor R115777 in patients with advanced breast cancer. *Proc Am Soc Clin Oncol* 2000; **83a**: Abstr 318